Urodynamics and Urinary Incontinence in Clinical Practice.

JORGE CLAVIJO EISELE. Editor.

Authors: Badia H, Chiba W, Craviotto F, Dieppa V, Mintegui D, Mouro L, Pou R, Rosenbaum T, Varela M.

Editor: Dr. J. Clavijo Eisele, FEBU. Profesor Agregado de Clínica Urológica. Facultad de Medicina. Univ. de la República. Montevideo. Uruguay. Consultant Urological Surgeon. St Hugh's Hospital. Grimsby. UK.

Invited authors: Badia H, Chiba W, Craviotto F, Dieppa V, Mintegui D, Mouro L, Pou R, Rosenbaum T, Varela M.

Proof: Dr A Presly, Mrs L Presly.

Print: CreateSpace. North Charleston, SC. USA.

Editorial: Urology Solutions Publishing.

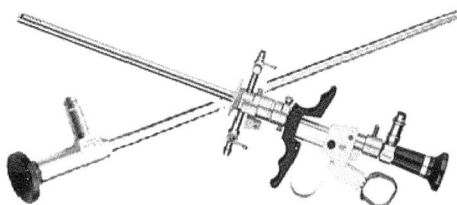

Urology Solutions Publishing

ISBN: 978-0-9931760-7-4

DEDICATION.

To the Urodynamics teams.
To the professionals who care for patients with incontinence and voiding dysfunctions.
To all our patients.

Mr. Jorge Clavijo-Eisele

TABLE OF CONTENTS.

INTRODUCTION.

You are at risk of having incontinence. We all are, even if we are in excellent health. Given the conditions (limits of physiological capacity) some trigger factors can lead anyone to an incontinence event. And that can be life changing, or at least very embarrassing. Continence is taken for granted, and when it's lost, it's perceived as a failure of the incontinent person in society, as it doesn't comply with general behavioural expectations. Humans don't become inured to incontinence well; it's always at least an "issue". Evolutionary, it's not useful to leave traces that can be tracked by your predators.

Urinary incontinence is a common symptom present in several disease conditions. It affects every population group, all ages and both sexes although it is more prevalent in females. It's an important health problem due to its frequency, severity, and psychological, social and economic impact. One in every 30 persons is incontinent. Women, the elderly, children and neurological patients have, as a consequence of their incontinence an objective medical and social problem and also a subjective psychological impact. All these usually lead to restriction in daily life activities. Work may need to be changed, socializing is restricted, dressing changes, the person may not be able to exercise or participate in sports, and sexual life may cease.

Today we can help incontinent patients. There are curative solutions in most occasions, either by diet and lifestyle interventions, medication, physical interventions, surgery or mostly by a combination of these. In some cases we have palliative strategies that can rescue patients from social isolation or exclusion. Always something can be done in spite of patient age. Benefits and risks of interventions have to be discussed in some detail and treatments have to be tailored to patients (and not patients accommodated into available treatments).

It is absolutely necessary that patients with urinary incontinence become co-responsible for their treatment and be proactive in their own care. This can be achieved by providing information and education to the patient and all those involved in his or her care including: social workers, nursing staff, doctors and everyone involved in the care of the incontinent patient.

Urodynamics and Urinary Incontinence in Clinical Practice.

Action speaks louder than words.

CHAPTER 1. PHYSIOLOGY OF CONTINENCE AND VOIDING.

Mouro L and Badia H.

VOIDING.

Voiding is a function of the lower urinary tract that results in the emptying of the bladder (Fig. 1). This normally happens when the bladder has reached its functional capacity and the situation is socially acceptable to do so.

Normal bladder function consists of two distinct phases: filling (storage or continence) phase and voiding (or emptying) phase.

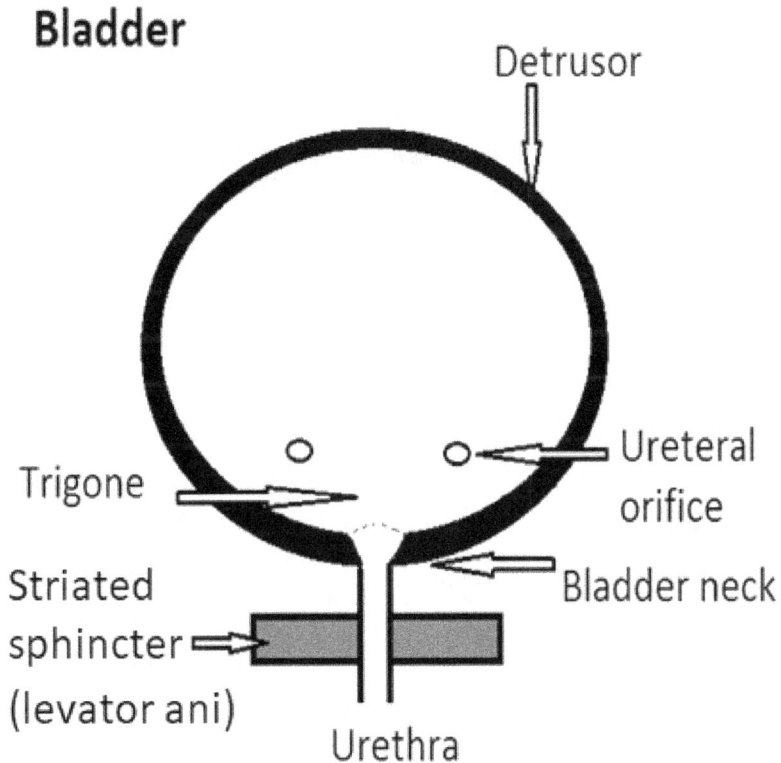

Fig. 1. Lower urinary tract. The space between the bladder neck and the sphincter is surrounded by the prostate in males.

Urinary incontinence is the consequence of a failure in the storage phase due to a urethral or bladder problem. Detrusor (bladder wall muscle) relaxation and urethral resting tone (urethral pressure) will determine continence. To understand the causes of incontinence it's useful to know how voiding happens.

During the filling phase the bladder relaxes and distends as the urine enters through the ureters (Fig. 2). The bladder has a round shape, is elastic and the filling process is usually unconscious. The urethra remains closed. The urethral closure mechanism includes the bladder neck (internal or smooth sphincter), the striated sphincter (peri-urethral fibres of the levator ani muscle, also known as pubococygeal) and the elastic fibres of the urethra itself that keep it passively collapsed.

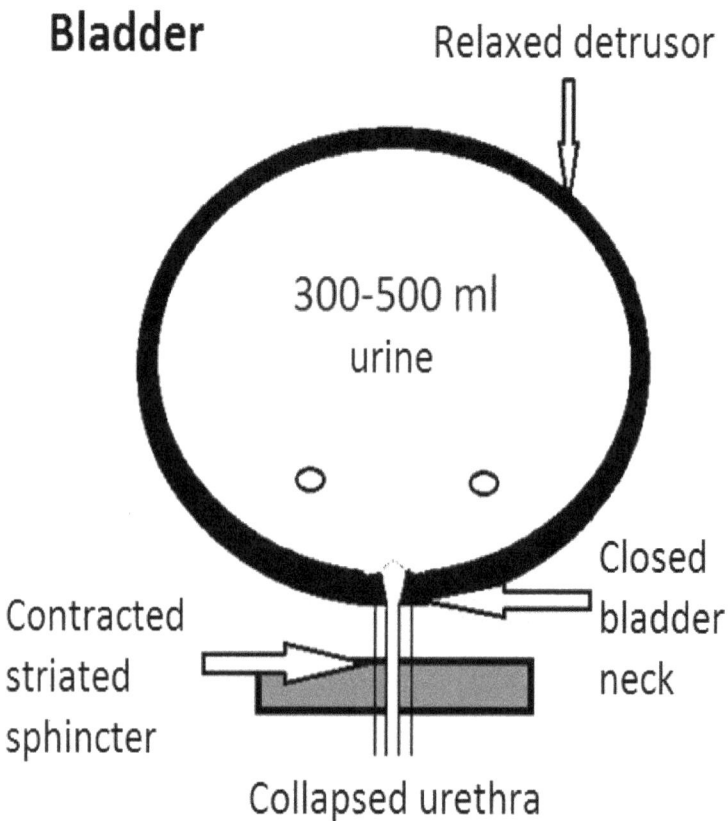

Fig. 2. Filling phase.

During the filling phase a person holds urine in the bladder for a period. This period is dependent on the rate of urine production (diuresis) and of social requirements (or mandates).

Diuresis depends on factors such as fluid intake, room temperature (and therefore perspiration), respiratory rate and physical activity. Bladder capacity is variable with most people having 350 to 500 ml (slightly larger in females). This capacity increases with age and is related to age and weight in children.

The bladder neck and striated sphincter remain closed during the filling phase whilst the detrusor accommodates to the increasing volume without any significant pressure rise inside the bladder.

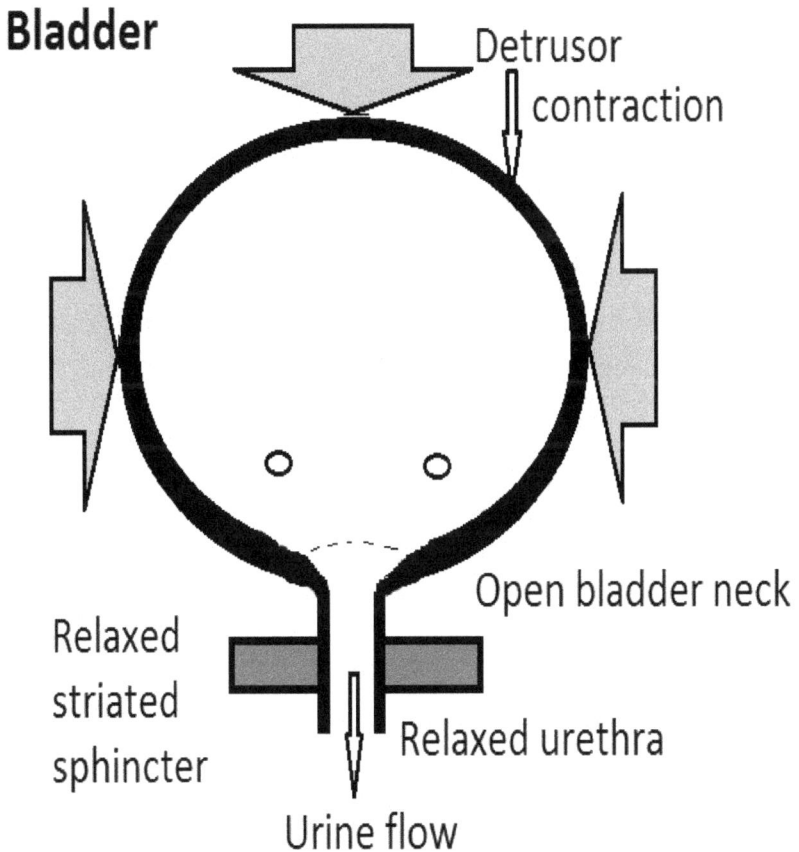

Fig. 3. Voiding phase.

When the bladder reaches its physiological capacity, and the person has no impediment (physical, psychological or social), then normal voiding can happen. In this emptying process the sphincter relaxes and the detrusor muscle contracts whilst the bladder neck opens and funnels (the proximal urethra opens) (Fig. 3).

Voiding is a voluntary and physiological action that requires co-ordination of the detrusor, bladder neck and striated sphincter. The relaxed urethra allows the passage of urine down to the meatus where it flows outwards due to the intra-vesical pressure generated by the detrusor contraction.

NEUROLOGICAL CONTROL OF VOIDING.

The nervous system controls the voiding cycle. Like with many other bodily systems, the nervous system regulates how the lower urinary tract functions. The filling or continence phase is involuntary and unconscious. It happens due to parasympathic control of the detrusor and sympathic control of the urethral closure system (bladder neck and striated sphincter mainly). Only if a person becomes aware of the possibility of leakage, the somatic voluntary nervous system participates in this control, by increasing the contraction of the striated sphincter, consequently increasing urethral resistance and therefore trying to prevent incontinence. The somatic voluntary nervous system is also used when the flow of urine is voluntarily interrupted (a non-physiological action, it can happen in reaction to a stimulus or unexpected dangerous or socially inconvenient situation during normal voiding- I am sure the reader can think of several examples of these faux pas).

The parasympathic nervous system has its medullary nuclei located in the sacral segments of the spinal cord (Fig. 4). The nerve from these nuclei is the pelvic plexus which innervates the detrusor and rest of the bladder, producing a detrusor contraction when activated. At the spinal level, the nucleus and nerve form a reflex arch with input through the dorsal fibres (afferent) and output through the ventral ones (efferent).

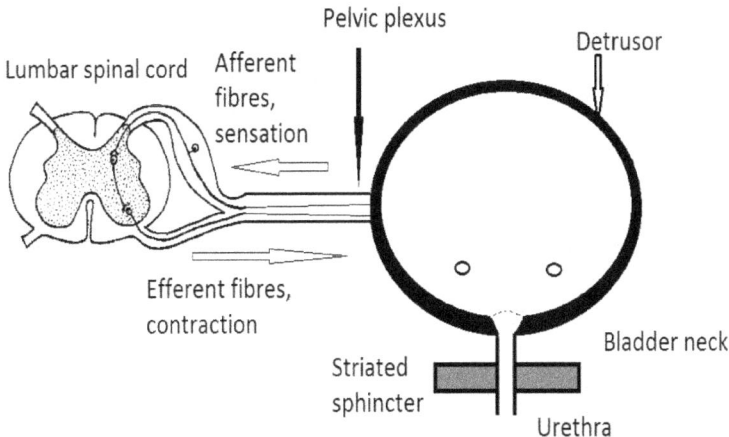

Fig. 4. Parasympathic system in the pelvis.

The sympathic nervous system has its medullary nuclei in the lower dorsal and upper lumbar segments of the spinal cord. The nerve is the hypogastric plexus. The sympathic action on the lower urinary tract is involuntary and it keeps a contraction tone on the bladder neck smooth muscle. This muscle tone keeps the bladder neck closed during the filling phase. There is some sympathic mediated relaxation of the detrusor as well during this phase.

The somatic nervous system has its medullary nuclei on the anterior horn of the sacral segments of the spinal cord (Onuf nucleus). The nerve is the pudendal nerve, which innervates the striated sphincter (levator ani or pubococygeal muscle). (Fig. 5).

These three nuclei and nerves are coordinated both during the filling and voiding phases. The coordination allows for normal function and for voluntary control from the cerebral cortex though the pontine micturition centre (Barrington's nucleus).

The nuclei that control voiding are:
- Sympathic: hypogastric plexus (T7-L1) innervates mainly the bladder neck (internal sphincter).
- Parasympathic: pelvis plexus (S2-S4) innervates mainly the detrusor.
- Somatic: pudendal nerve (S3-S4) innervates mainly the striated sphincter (levator ani).

The detrusor, due to its elastic fibres, accommodates (distends) during the filling phase, when there is a progressive increase of urine volume in the bladder without a significant rise in bladder pressure. This is why there is no sensation (initial voiding desire) until the bladder reaches its physiological distention capacity. When the bladder reaches its physiological functional capacity, the sensation of bladder fullness (need to void) travels through the sensitive fibres of the pelvic plexus to segments S2 to S4 of the spinal cord. At this level, the sensation enters through the posterior horns and reaches the parasympathic nucleus (in the intermedium-lateral horn). At this nucleus, the stimuli produce a motor response, which travels through the anterior horn and the efferent fibres of the pelvic plexus to the detrusor where it produces a contraction that will lead to the voiding phase.

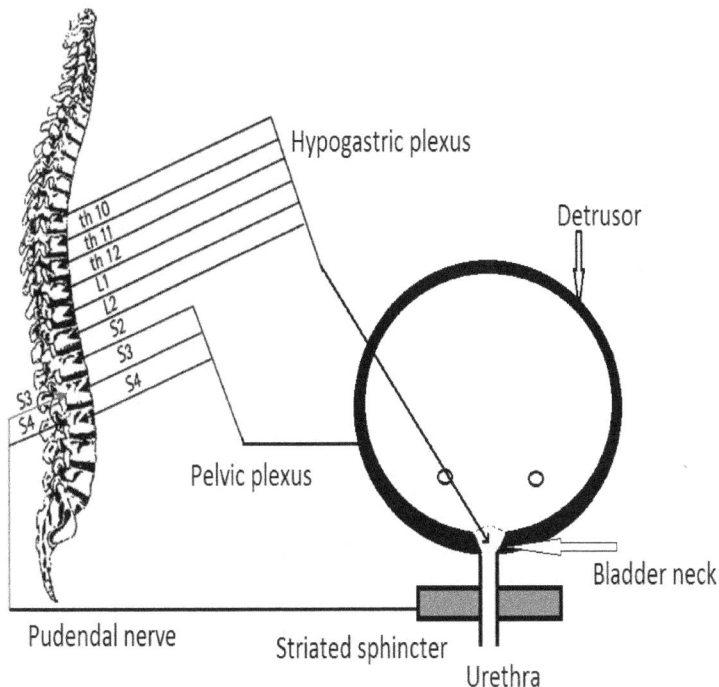

Fig. 5. Micturition control nuclei.

The parasympathic nucleus coordinates with the sympathic one, which turns off and relaxes the bladder neck (reduction in sympathic output). The detrusor, as a smooth muscle, contracts globally and progressively, rising the bladder pressure (normally below 40 cm H2O) and empties the bladder.

The striated sphincter has tonic fibres, which produce a basal muscle tone during the filling phase that closes the urethra. It also has phasic fibres that are only recruited as a response to the possibility of urine leakage or to try and stop the flow. The activity of the phasic fibres is voluntary and conscious.

When a small amount of urine enters the posterior urethra, the sensory fibres of the pudendal nerve take this information to the nucleus (at the anterior horn of the sacral spinal cord), where it produces a motor response. This will travel through the efferent fibres of this nerve to the phasic fibres of the sphincter that will contract. This contraction produces a very significant rise in the urethral closure pressure that prevents an unwanted urine leak.

These three nuclei must be co-ordinated and work synchronous to maintain a normal filling and voiding cycle.

During the filling phase (continence), there is a predominantly sympathic activity producing the bladder neck closure (alpha effect) and detrusor relaxation (beta effect); the parasympathic system is almost inactive, allowing for progressive detrusor distention. The pudendal nerve will only activate the phasic fibres of the sphincter if continence is threatened. Continence relies on sympathic activity. An additional active continence backup is provided by the phasic fibres of the pudendal nerve (in urgency) when there is a conscious sensation of imminent voiding.

The sequence of voiding includes the initial relaxation of the striated sphincter (tonic fibres) by a reduction of output (efferent) activity from the pudendal nucleus and nerve. This is followed by parasympathic activity (detrusor contraction) that occurs simultaneously to sympathic relaxation (bladder neck opening). The urethra needs to be open and with low resistance (closure pressure) before the detrusor contracts.

VOIDING COORDINATION.

During the filling phase the bladder neck and the striated sphincter remain closed to avoid urine leakage through the urethra. When the bladder has reached its functional capacity, before the detrusor contraction, the striated sphincter relaxes and the bladder neck opens at the time when the detrusor contraction begins. The required coordination of the medullary nuclei for a normal voiding takes place at the pontine micturition centre, or micturition coordination nucleus (Barrington centre). (Fig. 6).

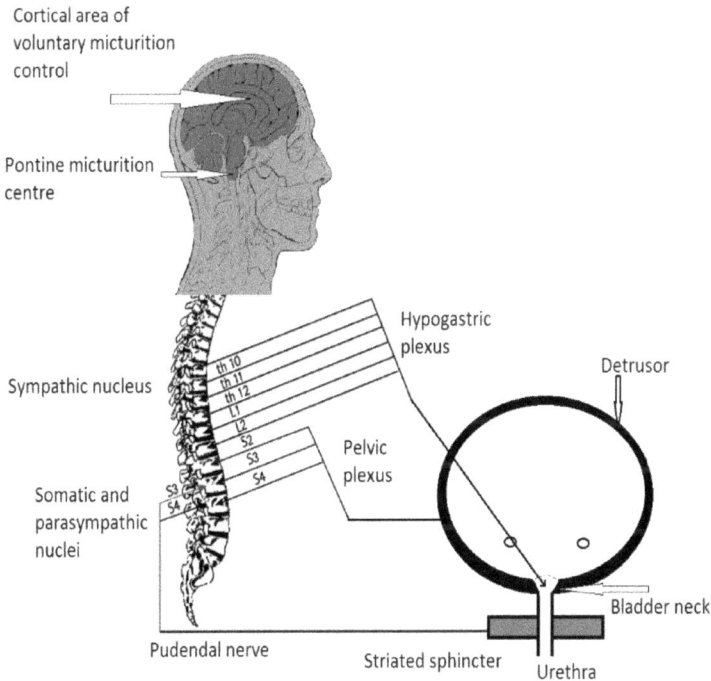

Fig. 6. Voiding coordination areas.

This coordination will prevent the medullary nuclei to work independently. Should this happen, a detrusor contraction could occur with the sphincter and bladder neck closed, producing an obstructive voiding. Alternatively the sphincter and bladder neck could open during the filling phase leading to incontinence. For this coordination to exist, it is necessary that all neurological

19

structures involved in continence and voiding are integrated and intact. Synchronicity is achieved through regulation (activation or inhibition) on the sympathic, parasympathic and pudendal nuclei by the pontine micturition centre in the brain stem. For an adequate function it is necessary the integrity of nerves and nuclei and also of the medullary pathways (in the spinal cord) that interconnect these nuclei (Fig. 7).

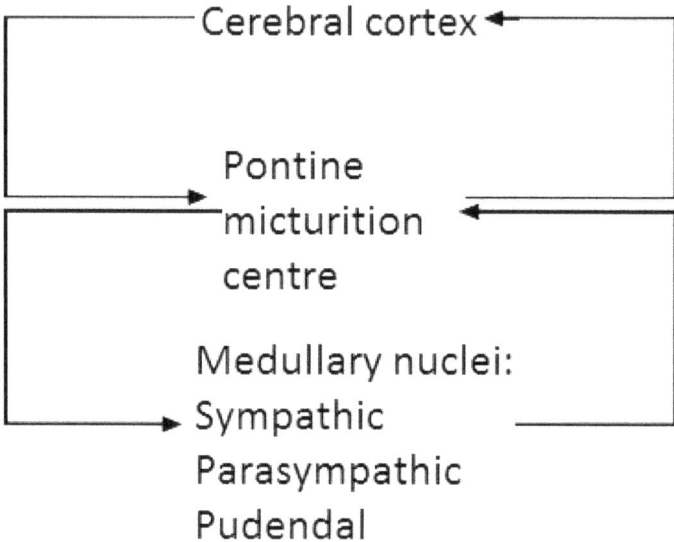

Cerebral cortex

Pontine
micturition
centre

Medullary nuclei:
Sympathic
Parasympathic
Pudendal

Fig. 7. Levels of voiding control.

The pontine micturition centre generates information that travels to the cerebral cortex conveying sensation of bladder volume. The need to void is controlled (postponed) by inhibiting the voiding reflex until voiding can take place in a convenient environment. Therefore, when circumstances are not adequate for voiding, in spite of a desire (perceived at the cortex), humans can willingly stop the voiding reflex. This happens as stimuli generated in the prefrontal cortex reach the pontine micturition centre, and this in turn inhibits the medullary nuclei preventing reflex voiding (Fig. 8). This system is immature in children before they can attain continence and damaged in several neurological conditions that present with incontinence.

Continence is the capacity of a person to differ voiding until emptying can take place in an adequate time and environment.

Cerebral cortex ↓ Voluntary control Pontine centre ↓ Coordination	Vertebrae	Spinal segments	Nerves	Targets
Sympathic nucleus	T7	T7-L1	Hypogastric plexus	Bladder neck
Parasympathic nucleus	T12-L1	S2-S4	Pelvic plexus	Detrusor

Fig. 8. Voluntary micturition control.

CONTINENCE MECANISMS.

To maintain continence the detrusor smooth muscle has to distend to accommodate a significant urine volume. The internal sphincter (bladder neck), urethral elasticity and coaptation and the slow twitch fibres of the striated sphincter prevent urine leakage. If an additional pressure is added to the bladder, the striated sphincter (fast twitch) and pelvic muscles help to maintain continence (by an additional increase in urethral resistance or closure pressure).

During the filling phase the urethral pressure (Pura) is higher than the bladder pressure (Pves), so the urine remains in the bladder. During voiding the urethral pressure lowers or ceases due to relaxation of the sphincters. The detrusor contracts and voiding ensues, since bladder pressure becomes higher than the urethral pressure. Incontinence happens when bladder pressure is higher than urethral pressure, which is when urethral closure pressure (UCP) is negative.

- UCP= urethral pressure (Pura) - bladder pressure (Pves)
- Bladder pressure (Pves) > urethral pressure (Pura) = voiding or incontinence
- Urethral pressure (Pura) > bladder pressure (Pves) = filling or retention

Ligaments failure, prolapse (hernia through the perineal hiatus) and pelvic muscles dysfunction in females lead to pelvic muscles and fascia becoming unable to prevent incontinence during stress manoeuvres (resting tone and phasic contraction are not effective). Bladder prolapse (cystocoele) and urethral prolapse (urethrocoele) change normal anatomy, so the affected structures lie outside (below) the area where an increase of urethral pressure would normally happen. If abdominal pressure (Pabd) rises due to a stress manoeuvre and the pressure is passed to the bladder (Pves) but not to the urethra (Pura), bladder pressure (Pves) will be higher than urethral pressure (Pura) and incontinence will happen.

Prolapse causes are varied (and debated), but it is a benign condition and in many cases preventable. Prolapse is an anatomical abnormality that needs to be repaired with or preferably before incontinence treatment. It is practically impossible to obtain normal function with abnormal anatomy, which is in line with the now fashionable integral theory.

In men, damage to the striated sphincter and its innervation (i.e. during prostate operations) produces lower muscle activity with reduced urethral pressure that may lead to incontinence.

MEMBRANE NEURO-RECEPTORS IN THE URINARY TRACT.

Synaptic transmission in the central, peripheral and autonomic nervous systems is mediated by neurotransmitters. It is quite relevant to know which are the neurotransmitters involved in the control of the lower urinary tract. This way we can use transmitter related medications to modify function as needed. Synaptic transmission in pre-ganglionic fibres in the sympathic and parasympathic systems is done by acetylcholine on nicotinic receptors.

Neuro-transmission between terminal axons (post-ganglionic) and smooth muscle is done by acetylcholine in the parasympathic system on muscarinic receptors. It is done by noradrenaline in the sympathic system on alpha (bladder neck) and beta receptors (detrusor). To differentiate on acetylcholine action on ganglia and muscle we use the terms nicotinic (ganglionic) and muscarinic (muscle). The response to noradrenaline is not always the same, in some cases it produces contraction (alpha receptors on the bladder neck) and in others relaxation (beta receptors on the detrusor), these different responses are due to the different receptors' activities (Fig. 9).

The receptors located in the cells of the bladder wall, bladder neck and striated sphincter are cell specific molecules that bind to neurotransmitters and interact with them producing a pre-determined response in the cell.

The bladder cells have several receptors that can be modified by medications. The most relevant ones regarding voiding and continence are adrenergic and cholinergic receptors. The distribution of receptors includes: parasympathic cholinergic receptors and beta adrenergic ones are located mainly on the bladder wall and detrusor muscle. Alpha adrenergic receptors are mainly located at the bladder neck, bladder base and proximal urethra (Fig. 10).

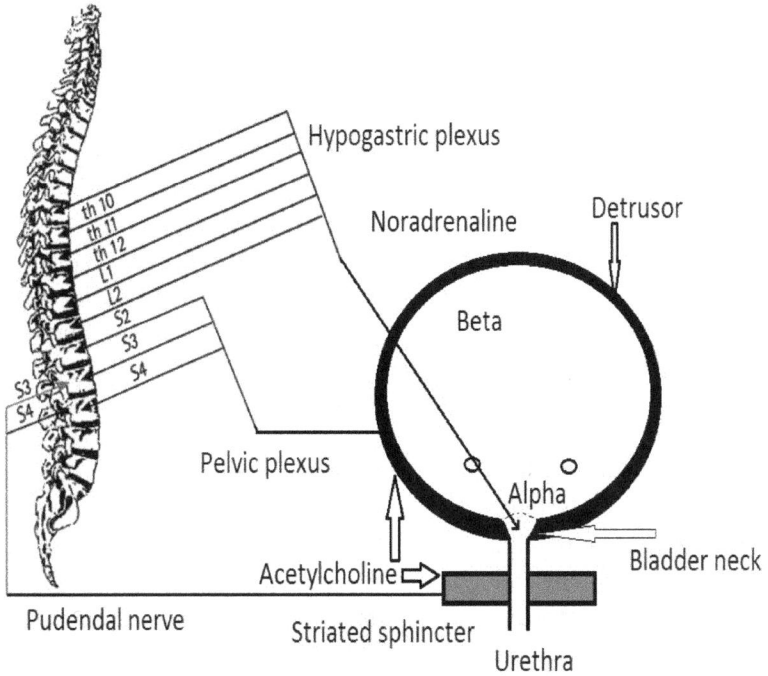

Fig. 9. Receptors distribution in the lower urinary tract.

Cholinergic receptors are present in the whole bladder and urethra but are particularly numerous on the bladder wall.

ORGAN AREA	RECEPTORS	ACTION
Detrusor	Cholinergic muscarinic	Detrusor contraction
Detrusor	Beta adrenergic	Detrusor relaxation
Bladder neck	Alpha adrenergic	Bladder neck contraction
Striated sphincter	Cholinergic nicotinic	Striated sphincter contraction

Fig. 10. Receptors distribution and action in the lower urinary tract.

CONTINENCE DEVELOPMENT.

During the first year of life voiding is triggered not only when the bladder reaches its physiological capacity but also with any external stimuli capable of inducing detrusor reflex contraction with the relaxation of the bladder neck and striated sphincter. Even under these premises some studies have shown that the central nervous system also participates in sphincter control since the foetal stage. It has been found that in new-borns the bladder is generally relaxed, and they don't urinate during sleep. This detrusor inhibition during sleep has been found even in children with daytime bladder over activity.

In the period of life before voluntary bladder control, voiding is generally automatic, involuntary and coordinated. At this stage there is no myelinisation of the control pathways from the cerebral cortex to the pontine micturition centre (PMC - Barrington's coordination nucleus). The PMC works normally, but it is unregulated by the cerebral cortex.

Voiding pressures are higher in children than in adults. There are also differences between the sexes: males reach voiding pressures of 118 cm H2O and females 75 cm H2O on average. These pressures lower with age. Video-urodynamics have also shown that up to 70% of 3 year old children have intermittent voiding patterns that tend to disappear with age. These facts seem to mirror the progressive development stages in detrusor–sphincter coordination.

Between the first and second years of life children develop the conscious sensation of bladder fullness. The capacity to empty the bladder or prevent a bladder contraction at different volumes of filling is generally developed during the third year of life. Cerebral cortex inhibition over the PMC is crucial to achieve continence. Through an active learning process, the child develops the will to inhibit or postpone voiding until it is considered acceptable. From birth until adult voiding patterns are reached an intact nervous system is necessary to control the lower urinary tract and obtain a progressive increase in bladder capacity. This stage is usually reached between 3 and 5 years, when children become continent during the day and finally also at night.

Voiding control is complex and involves several areas through the central, peripheral and autonomic nervous systems and the urinary tract.

Incontinence at night is called enuresis. It is still present in 20% of children at 4 years and 10% of children by 8 years.

URINARY INCONTINENCE (UI).

Urinary incontinence is the involuntary leakage of urine.

This produces a hygienic, social and psychological problem for the sufferer and a significant limitation to his/her work activity, education and personal life. This problem affects all ages and both sexes. It has similar incidence in childhood, and becomes more prevalent in females in adult life. After 65 years the prevalence of incontinence rises significantly and becomes proportional to age. Sex differences tend to remain the same or decrease at this stage.

Incontinence is not a disease in itself, but a consequence of an alteration of the bladder's filling phase. It can be present in several diseases, where it is both a symptom and a sign. Incontinence can be:
- A symptom: the patient refers urine leakage.
- A sign: it is the objective demonstration of urine loss.
- A physiological alteration: the urodynamic evidence of incontinence and its cause.

Incontinence as a symptom:
- Urge urinary incontinence: is the involuntary leak of urine associated to an intense desire to void (urgency).
- Stress urinary incontinence: the patient refers as a symptom involuntary leakage related to movements and manoeuvres that increase intra-abdominal pressure (cough, strain, laugh, and sneeze).
- Unaware incontinence: leakage happens in absence of urgency or stress manoeuvres and without conscious recognition of the leakage.
- Enuresis: the term is used to describe incontinence during sleep.
- Post-void incontinence or dribbling: leakage after normal voiding.
- Continuous incontinence: permanent leakage, usually of small amounts.

Incontinence as a sign:

Urine loss can be seen during stress manoeuvres or movement in stress incontinence (ask patient to cough or squeeze the abdomen in the Valsalva manoeuvre). Post void incontinence and continuous incontinence are easily identifiable. **Extra urethral urinary incontinence is the clinical diagnosis of a urinary fistula.**

Incontinence as an urodynamic finding:
Clinical tests and specially urodynamic studies (UDS) can show where the incontinence cause is located in the lower urinary tract.

- Stress incontinence: happens when, without detrusor contraction, bladder pressure (Pves) is higher than urethral pressure (Pura). The diagnosis is incompetence of the urethral closure system (or mechanism).
- Overactive detrusor incontinence: happens during an involuntary contraction (IC) of the detrusor during the filling phase (urodynamic detrusor over activity, UDO). It is generally related to urgency, in which case it can also be called urge incontinence (UI).
- Overflow incontinence: happens due to bladder hiper-distention. By definition it is a complete urinary retention.

Incontinence is a consequence of a disease, and not a disease state in itself. This definition creates a problem for its study and treatment. There is ongoing discussion at the WHO to recognize incontinence as a disease and not as an alteration of normal health which is the present situation.

Aetiology of urinary incontinence:
Causes of overactive detrusor include:

- Idiopathic over activity if there is no demonstrable neurological cause.
- Neurogenic hyperactivity or hyper-reflexia in the presence of neurological disease.
- Bladder irritation and inflammation by infectious, cancerous, chemical, radiation and mechanical sources.

Causes of incompetence of the urethral closure system:

- Striated sphincter and pelvic muscles failure by neurological or muscle damage.

- Failure of bladder neck due to inappropriate relaxation or anatomical lesion.
- Lack of urethral coaptation. In women, intrinsic urethral sphincter deficiency is commonly associated with multiple anti-incontinence surgical procedures, as well as with hypo-oestrogenism and aging. Patients often leak continuously or with minimal exertion. During cystoscopy the urethra may be shortened, with an open bladder neck, a short striated sphincter area which doesn't contract much when asking the patient to cough. The urethra may have lost its elastic capacity to close when the cystoscope has the fluid stopped giving the rigid, non-collapsible "lead pipe" view. Similar findings can be elicited by a well conducted cysto-urethrogram. In urodynamic studies it is a severe form of stress urinary incontinence, equating it to type III stress urinary incontinence defined as a Valsalva leak point pressure of less than 60 cm H2O.
- Lack of normal urethral support during stress manoeuvres.

3. Combination of the above.

Terminology.
The International Continence Society has produced documents with recommended definitions which are useful most of the time (ICS) and facilitate standardisation.

Lower urinary tract symptoms (LUTS).
Symptoms are subjective. They are related by the patient, family members or carers and they may be the reason for seeking care. Symptoms can also be elicited during consultation.

Storage symptoms include:
Frequency: patient perception that the frequency of voiding is increased. Polaquiuria.
Nocturia: waking up to void during the night.
Urgency: sudden appearance of a desire to void which is difficult to postpone.
Urinary incontinence: the patient refers a urine leak. Relevant factors include type, frequency, severity, triggers, social impact, effect on hygiene and quality of life, measures used to handle the incontinence and whether the patient wants help or not with the

condition. Stress, urge, mixed or continuous type of incontinence. There are unusual types of incontinence such as incontinence during sex and giggle incontinence. Functional incontinence is the term used to describe leakage unrelated to abnormalities of the urinary tract or nervous system, the typical example being incontinence due to reduced mobility (cannot reach a facility in time). (Fig. 11).

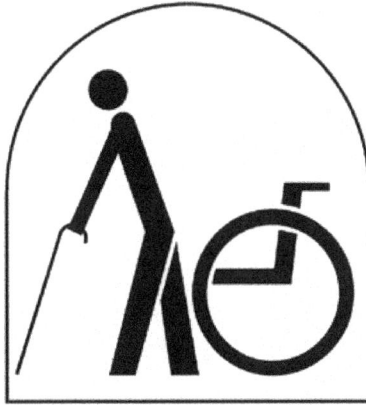

Fig. 11. Restricted mobility may lead to functional incontinence. Voiding symptoms (emptying), like slow and or weak flow, intermittent flow, straining, hesitancy and incomplete emptying sensation (tenesmus) can present alongside incontinence.

Signs suggestive of lower urinary tract dysfunction.
Signs are objective indicators of disease as observed by a healthcare provider, including simple manoeuvres to verify and quantify the symptoms. Voiding diaries (frequency/volume charts), number of pads (or other protection used) and validated questionnaires of symptoms and quality of life (IPSS, AUASI, ICIQ, UDI-6, etc.) are examples of instruments that need to be used to verify and quantify symptoms (Fig. 12 to 14).

Syndromes from lower urinary tract dysfunction.
Syndromes are groups of symptoms and signs that suggest a particular dysfunction or anatomical change. The most frequent ones include:
- Overactive bladder (OAB) syndrome: urgency, frequency, nocturia and sometimes urge incontinence. This syndrome is

suggestive of detrusor hyperactivity (involuntary detrusor contractions during the filling phase).

- Voiding syndrome (formerly prostatism): voiding symptoms as described above usually associated with an obstructive pattern in a flow measurement with or without post micturition residual.

ADDITIONAL READING.

1. The integral system. Petros P. Cent European J Urol. 2011; 64(3):110-9.
2. The prevalence of urinary incontinence. Nitti VW. Rev Urol. 2001;3 Suppl 1:S2-6.
3. Urinary incontinence: useful concepts for primary care. (Incontinencia urinaria: conceptos útiles para Atención Primaria). Martínez Agulló E, Albert Torne R, Bernabé Corral B. Indas; 1998. p.19-42.
4. The standardisation of terminology of lower urinary tract function: report from the Standardisation Sub-committee of the International Continence Society. Abrams P, Cardozo L, Fall M, et al. Neurourol Urodyn 2002; 21(2): 167-78.
5. Giggle incontinence. Fernández, W., Clavijo, J. Lab. de Neuro-urología. Depto. de Urología. Hosp. de Clínicas. Montevideo. I Congreso Ibero-Americano de Neuro-urología y Uro-ginecología. Punta Del Este. Uruguay. 1989.
6. Urinary incontinence (Incontinencia Urinaria). Fernandez-Gomez W, Pereyra-Flores W, Costabel G, Clavijo J, Nallem J, Montero D. Cuad. Urol. Urug. p. 1-5, 1993.

Useful forms:

Urogenital Distress Inventory - Short Form (UDI-6)

Do you experience and, if so, how much are you bothered by:	Not at all	Slightly	Moderately	Greatly
Frequent urination?	0	1	2	3
Urine leakage related to the feeling of urgency?	0	1	2	3
Urine leakage related to physical activity, coughing, or sneezing?	0	1	2	3
Small amounts of urine leakage (drops)?	0	1	2	3
Difficulty emptying your bladder?	0	1	2	3
Pain or discomfort in the lower abdominal or genital area?	0	1	2	3

Symptom score _____

Fig. 14. UDI-6 form.[i]

Name_____Date_____

Use the diary below to record urinary output, fluids consumed, and urinary leakage (if applicable) for 3 complete 24-hour periods. If you used a catheter to empty your bladder, record those volumes in the specified column.

Time of day (circle bedtime and wake up times below; also fill in events at right in time slots when they occurred)	Fluid Intake (write down amount of liquid you drank (in oz) from toileting event to next)	Toilet Urinations (write down oz urinated into urinary hat each time you urinate)	Amount of urine drained via cathether (if using a catheter, record amount (in oz, ml, or cc; indicate catheter [C] or residual {R}	Leaks (place check mark in column if you leaked urine before making it to the toilet)	Pad Changes (at each toileting event, write "D" if pad was dry or "W" if pad was wet; write if amount was small, mod, or large)
7 am					
8 am					
9 am					
10 am					
11 am					
Noon					
1 pm					
2 pm					
3 pm					
4 pm					
5 pm					
6 pm					
7 pm					
8 pm					
9 pm					
10 pm					
11 pm					
Midnight					
1 am					
2 am					
3 am					
4 am					
5 am					
6 am					

Fig. 12. Voiding diary.[ii]

International Prostate Symptom Score (I-PSS)

Patient Name: _____ Date of birth: _____ Date completed _____

In the past month:	Not at All	Less than 1 in 5 Times	Less than Half the Time	About Half the Time	More than Half the Time	Almost Always	Your score
1. Incomplete Emptying How often have you had the sensation of not emptying your bladder?	0	1	2	3	4	5	
2. Frequency How often have you had to urinate less than every two hours?	0	1	2	3	4	5	
3. Intermittency How often have you found you stopped and started again several times when you urinated?	0	1	2	3	4	5	
4. Urgency How often have you found it difficult to postpone urination?	0	1	2	3	4	5	
5. Weak Stream How often have you had a weak urinary stream?	0	1	2	3	4	5	
6. Straining How often have you had to strain to start urination?	0	1	2	3	4	5	
	None	1 Time	2 Times	3 Times	4 Times	5 Times	
7. Nocturia How many times did you typically get up at night to urinate?	0	1	2	3	4	5	
Total I-PSS Score							

Score: 1-7: *Mild*   8-19: *Moderate*   20-35: *Severe*

Quality of Life Due to Urinary Symptoms	Delighted	Pleased	Mostly Satisfied	Mixed	Mostly Dissatisfied	Unhappy	Terrible
If you were to spend the rest of your life with your urinary condition just the way it is now, how would you feel about that?	0	1	2	3	4	5	6

Fig. 13. IPSS symptom score[iii].

CHAPTER 2. DIAGNOSIS OF URINARY INCONTINENCE.

Pou R and Clavijo J.

UI is the involuntary leakage of urine through the urethra, which can be objectively identified and produces a social and/or hygienic problem.

The diagnostic pathway needs to be systematic, as diagnosis will determine which treatment will be recommended. UI is more prevalent in women, increasing with age, in later life the incidence tends to equalize.

Prevalence of UI.
Sex:
- Females 16,1%
- Men 14,5%

Age:
- 65-74 years 13,3%
- 75-84 years 16,3%
- 84 years 26,3%

The classic groups affected by incontinence are:
- Enuretic children.

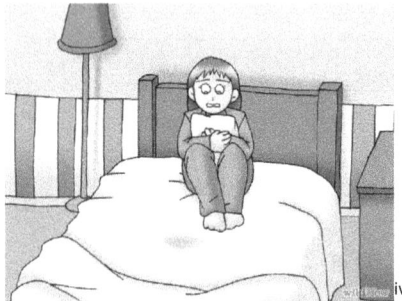

Fig. 15. Enuretic children have a family impact.

- Multiparous adult females of working age.

- Geriatric adults of both sexes affected by bladder dysfunction, mobility and urine production problems.
- Neurological patients with neurogenic bladder dysfunction secondary to Parkinson's, cerebral-vascular accident (CVA), spinal cord injury (SCI), multiple sclerosis (MS), and other neurological diseases.

UI has several risk factors that may lead to its onset. Some can be improved or eliminated to restore continence completely or partially. (Fig. 16).

UI risk factors.
Modifiable factors:
- Prolapse.
- Urinary infection.
- Constipation and other bowel dysfunctions.
- Smoking, alcoholism.
- Obesity.
- Medications.
- Co-morbidities like diabetes, hypertension and COPD.
- Other conditions that increase intra-abdominal pressure.
- High caffeine intake.

Non-modifiable factors:
- Age.
- Previous vaginal deliveries.
- Hysterectomy.
- Menopause.
- Previous pelvic surgery.
- Neurological lesions.

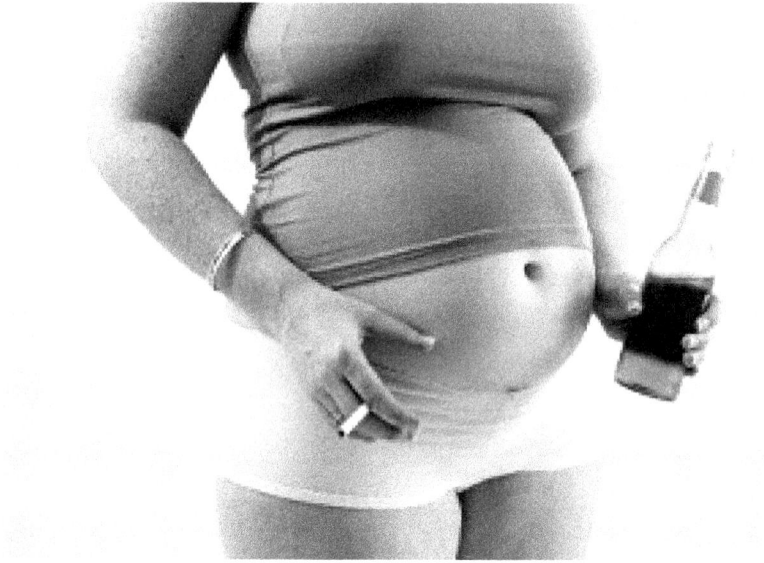

Fig. 16. UI risk factors: female sex, white race, pregnancies and vaginal deliveries, smoking, alcoholism, obesity.

CLINICAL CLASSIFICATION.

Four clinical types of incontinence account for the vast majority of cases: stress incontinence, urge incontinence, mixed incontinence and overflow incontinence (Fig. 17a). An initial idea of the type can be obtained from the ICIQ form.

Stress UI.
It is leakage produced by an increase in intra-abdominal pressure such as cough, laughter, the Valsalva manoeuvre, sneezing or any other physical effort. It happens due to a failure of the urethral closure system with normal detrusor activity. There is usually no previous desire to void. It's the most frequent type in females. Predisposing factors are obesity, pregnancies and vaginal deliveries, muscle relaxant medication, smoking, COPD, neurological diseases (particularly peripheral neuropathies) and oestrogen deficit in postmenopausal life.

Urge UI.
It's leakage preceded by an intense and sudden desire to void, of which the patient is conscious about. In many cases the leakage happens on the way to the toilet. It is usually due to involuntary detrusor contractions, which can be registered in an urodynamic study. Predisposing factors are neurological diseases (Parkinson's, Alzheimer, CVAs, MS, etc.), previous urological operations, urological diseases (stones, infections), stool impaction, diverticulitis. Urgency with or without frequency is called overactive bladder and it implies more than 9 voids per day with normal diuresis (daily urine production).

Mixed UI.
It's involuntary urine leakage with symptoms of both stress and urge incontinence. It's due to combined detrusor over activity and dysfunction of the urethral closure system. It's frequently seen in elderly females and older males with voiding symptoms.

Overflow UI.
It is leakage caused by an over distended bladder, with a bladder pressure (Pves) higher than the Urethral pressure (Pura). The

urethral closure system is usually intact (bladder neck and sphincter). Two processes lead to it:

- Sub-vesical obstruction, like an enlarged prostate.
- Detrusor failure during voiding, like detrusor muscle damage, peripheral neuropathy or medications' side effects.

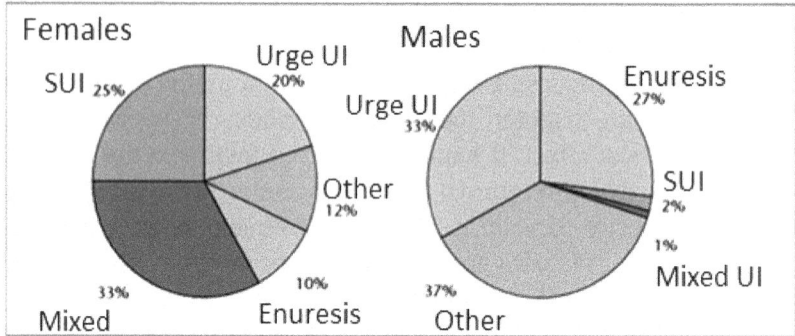

Fig. 17a. Types of UI by sex. From Carretero-Colmer M.

There are other clinical types of incontinence but are far less frequent, like **transient urinary incontinence** seen in the elderly (Fig. 17b). This is due to specific trigger factors including: delirium, infection of urine, atrophy of the vagina, multi-medication, psychological problems, excess of urine production, restriction in mobility and stool impaction (DIAPPERS). Other infrequent types include **giggle incontinence, coital incontinence and orgasmic incontinence (climacturia)**.

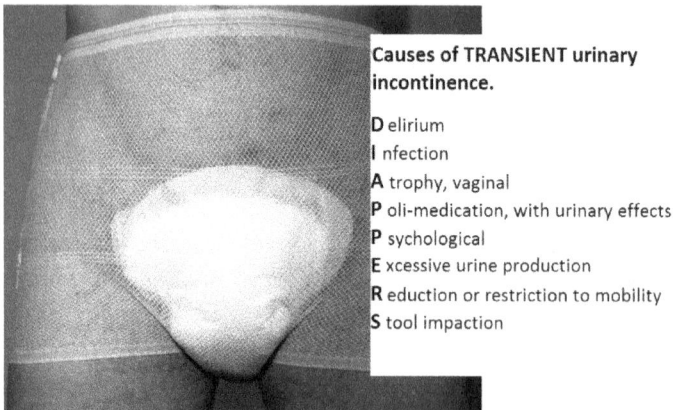

Causes of TRANSIENT urinary incontinence.

D elirium
I nfection
A trophy, vaginal
P oli-medication, with urinary effects
P sychological
E xcessive urine production
R eduction or restriction to mobility
S tool impaction

Fig. 17b. Transient urinary incontinence causes.

40

CLINICAL DIAGNOSIS.

The clinical diagnosis of UI is a process that can be done in primary care by a trained professional. History taking has to be specific and focused and can be greatly aided by the use of the above mentioned questionnaires (ICIQ). Sometimes incontinence may not be the main reason for an appointment, but the condition will surface when asked, and usually explains much of the patient's situation.

— History: general, focused, IPSS (males), ICIQ and 3 day voiding diary.
— Examination: general, gynaecologic, rectal exam, focused neurological in some cases. Stress test: standing on a piece of paper, with legs separated, stress manoeuvre (Fig. 18).

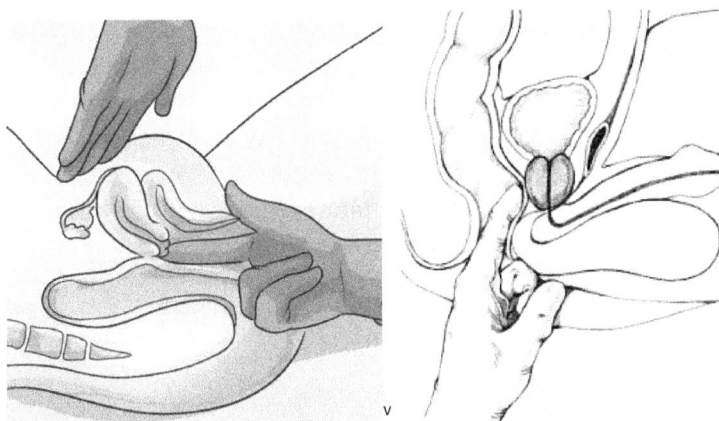

Fig. 18. Pelvic female and male examinations.

— Laboratory exams.
— Imaging tests.
— Additional tests, particularly cystoscopy and urodynamics (UDS).

General history.
Every diagnosis starts with good history taking. Sex, age, smoking and alcohol consumption needs recording. It's important to know the function of the digestive system, particularly constipation or faecal incontinence. Calculate BMI or abdominal perimeter to assess the degree of obesity. In females register menopausal

41

status or type of cycles as well as parity. Past history may show neurological conditions, diabetes or skeletal problems affecting walking and mobility. Check previous operations, particularly in the pelvis, lower abdomen or spine. Inquire about sexual function. Check above mentioned risk factors.

Focused history.
Check when UI began and under which circumstances. Was there any relevant health event like surgery, CVA, new medication, new diagnosis, delivery, etc.? Always check in the elderly for transient incontinence triggers. Ask the patient the impact incontinence has on life activities as well as number of UI events and estimated amount (volume) of leakage. Ask the patient to complete an ICIQ before or after the initial consultation (Fig. 19). Try to find triggers like stress, laughter, cold or hearing or touching water. Ask if leakage is preceded by a desire to void. Check time of the day and night that UI happens. Ask how it happens (post void dribble, continuous, intermittent, etc.). Use standard tools like the UDI and a 3 to 5 day voiding diary. This gives useful information on probable aetiology, severity and frequency of the UI. Ask about gynaecologic and obstetric history, number of deliveries, need for instrumentation (forceps), complications, episiotomy, sutures, new-born weight, pelvic surgery and menopause.

ICIQ-UI Short Form

Initial number

CONFIDENTIAL

Today's date

DAY MONTH YEAR

Many people leak urine some of the time. We are trying to find out how many people leak urine, and how much this bothers them. We would be grateful if you could answer the following questions, thinking about how you have been, on average, over the PAST FOUR WEEKS.

1 **Please write in your date of birth:**

DAY MONTH YEAR

2 **Are you** *(tick one)*: Female Male

3 **How often do you leak urine?** *(Tick one box)*

never	0
about once a week or less often	1
two or three times a week	2
about once a day	3
several times a day	4
all the time	5

4 **We would like to know how much urine you think leaks.**
How much urine do you usually leak (whether you wear protection or not)?
(Tick one box)

none	0
a small amount	2
a moderate amount	4
a large amount	6

5 **Overall, how much does leaking urine interfere with your everyday life?**
Please ring a number between 0 (not at all) and 10 (a great deal)

0 1 2 3 4 5 6 7 8 9 10
not at all   a great deal

ICIQ score: sum scores 3+4+5

6 **When does urine leak?** *(Please tick all that apply to you)*

never – urine does not leak	
leaks before you can get to the toilet	
leaks when you cough or sneeze	
leaks when you are asleep	
leaks when you are physically active/exercising	
leaks when you have finished urinating and are dressed	
leaks for no obvious reason	
leaks all the time	

Thank you very much for answering these questions.

Copyright © "ICIQ Group"

vi

Fig. 19. ICIQ form. The ICIQ form is useful, validated and easily filled by the patient. Quality of life is measured adding answers to questions 3 to 5. The higher the score, the worse the quality. Sequential use can measure the result of treatment interventions.

Carefully note medications used. Most incontinent patients are elderly and take many medications, several of which may have direct or secondary effects on the urinary tract. Yet, before ascribing incontinence on a medication we must rule out other frequent causes (Fig. 20).

CLASS	MEDICATION	EFFECT
Anticholinergics	Atropine, hyoscine	Detrusor relaxation
Sedatives, anxiolytics, sleep medication	Benzodiazepines	Relaxation of striated sphincter, reduced mobility
Diuretics	Furosemide, thiazides	Increased diuresis
Alpha blockers	Tamsulosin, alfuzosin, doxazosin, clonidine	Relaxation of bladder neck
ACEI	Enalapril, captopril	Cough
Antidepressants	Imipramine, paroxetine, fluoxetine	Detrusor relaxation, bladder neck closure
Antipsychotics	Haloperidol, quetiapine, chlorpromazine	Detrusor relaxation, sedation, reduced mobility
Anti-histaminic	Promethazine, chlorpheniramine	Detrusor relaxation, sedation, reduced mobility
Calcium channel blockers	Nifedipine, amlodipine	Detrusor relaxation
Adrenergics	Ephedrine, terbutaline, salbutamol, phenylephrine	Detrusor relaxation, bladder neck closure, increased tone of striated sphincter
Opiates	Morphine, tramadol, codeine	Detrusor relaxation, sedation, reduced mobility
Muscle relaxants	Tizanidine, baclofen, dantrolene	Relaxation of striated sphincter, reduced mobility

Fig. 20. Some medications and their effects on continence.

Whenever it's possible (and this is infrequent), we can try to change medications and see if continence improves.

Physical exam.
This is the most variable part of the consultation. Ideally a full complete exam should be carried out. On real life clinical practice this is rarely possible or needed. Observe the patient as he/she walks in the room, do they have gait problems? Uses sticks? Short-sighted? Significant obesity? Check manual dexterity and sight in patients that may require intermittent catheterisation. Explore the abdomen for a palpable bladder, abdominal or pelvic masses that can compress the bladder. Gynaecological exam looking for prolapse, degree and type, atrophy and urethral mobility. During palpation, assess perineal muscles tone. Standing, perform the stress test as described below (Fig. 21). In males do rectal examination; assess perineal muscles tone and prostate. Rectal examination (DRE) provides information of stool impaction, and bulbo-cavernous reflex (checks integrity of reflex arc in S2-S4).

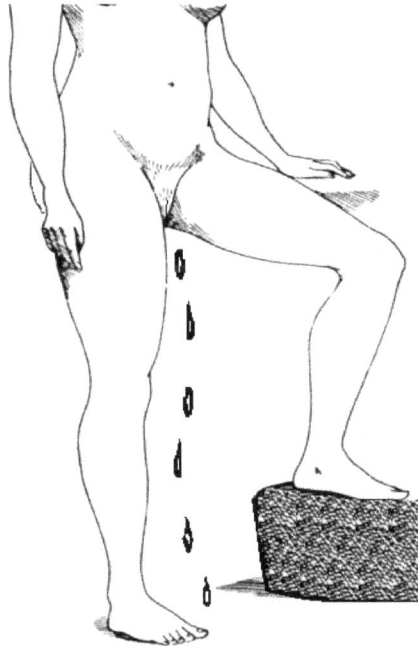

Fig. 21. Perform stress test and check for prolapse in standing position.

Assess cognitive function in neurological patients.

Lab tests.
Usually renal function and glycaemia are checked. A urine dip test can show signs of infection (and then a urine culture would be required), it will also show pH, density and suspicion of haematuria. All patients with catheters or external drainages will be colonized by bacteria. In these cases **do not do urine test nor urine culture** (only blood culture if there is fever or intense pyuria). (Fig. 22).

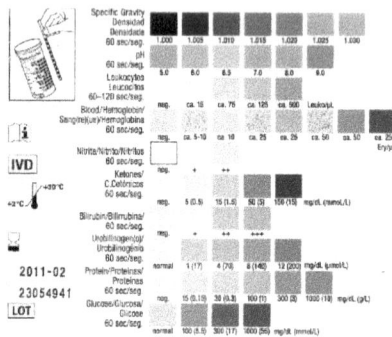

Fig. 22. Urine dip test kit.

Imaging tests.
Assess bladder post void residual, which becomes significant when > 50 ml (or > 10% of maximum bladder capacity). A simple method is using an automated scan. More precise but more invasive is catheterising the patient and measuring the obtained volume. An ultrasound scan of the urinary tract will inform the residual. The ultrasound scan (USS) is also useful to check for abnormalities in the urinary tract, renal alterations and to measure the prostate volume.

Additional tests.
In many cases where there is the possibility of a problem (congenital or acquired) of the lower urinary tract, a **cystoscopy** is indicated. This allows checking for urethral lesions, fistulae, compressions, stones, diverticula, tumours, strictures and other abnormalities that may predispose to incontinence.

The most precise technique to study incontinence are **urodynamic studies (UDS)**, which assess lower urinary tract function during the filling and voiding phases. This is done by recording urinary pressures, flow and volume. This study is generally useful to differentiate stress from urge incontinence. It is indicated in those patients with previous pelvic surgical procedures, neurological patients, patients with suspicion of associated voiding obstruction, or clinically unclear cases. Do not perform UDS before starting conservative (non-surgical) management. The detailed technique will be described later (Fig. 23).

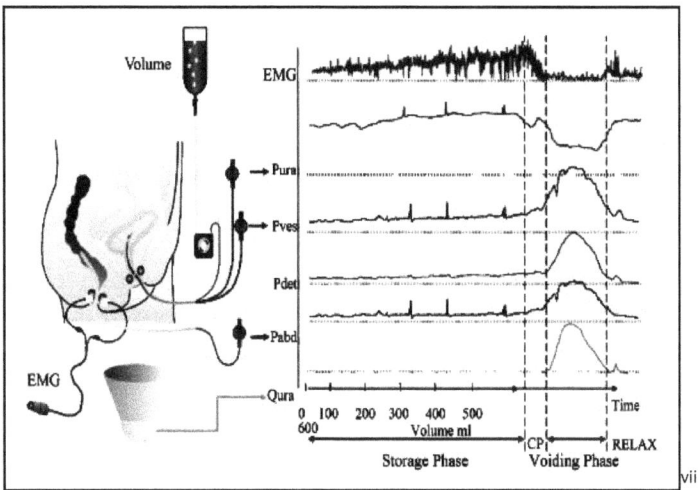

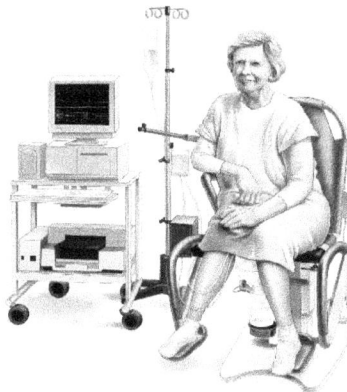

Fig. 23. UDS in a female.

There are several UDS, the most frequent measurements used are: flow rate, cystometry (with leak pressures) and pressure-flow studies.

- Flow rate is the measurement of the urinary output in physiological conditions (usually sitting in females and standing in males). A high flow in a short time indicates a likely easy void and is frequently seen in stress incontinence.
- Cystometry is the record of pressures during the filling phase, usually in the bladder and abdomen (with a rectal sensor). The filling is done at a controlled rate. If there is leakage, the pressure at that point is registered.
- Pressure-flow studies is the record of the same pressures during the voiding phase.

Pves is measured with a bladder catheter. Pabd by a rectal catheter. Detrusor pressure (Pdet) is calculated by the data processor (computer) as Pves-Pabd. Flow rate is recorded by a flowmeter under the patient during incontinence or at the voiding (micturition) command. If there is suspicion of a neurological disorder, an electro-myogram of the pubococygeal muscle (levator ani, or striated sphincter) is recorded usually by means of skin (surface) electrodes.

Under normal conditions, during the filling phase, the detrusor muscle does not have any significant contractile activity (it actually relaxes). Pves does not rise, and there is a progressive sensation of bladder filling (stable detrusor). If there are involuntary detrusor contractions (IDC) during the filling phase (urodynamic detrusor over activity, UDO), the bladder pressure rises, and it usually produces urgency with or without urinary incontinence. IDC are a transient increase in Pdet during the filling phase. The classic definition is an increase of > 15 cm H2O for over 15 seconds, but any increase in bladder pressure in the filling phase can explain symptoms (Fig. 24).

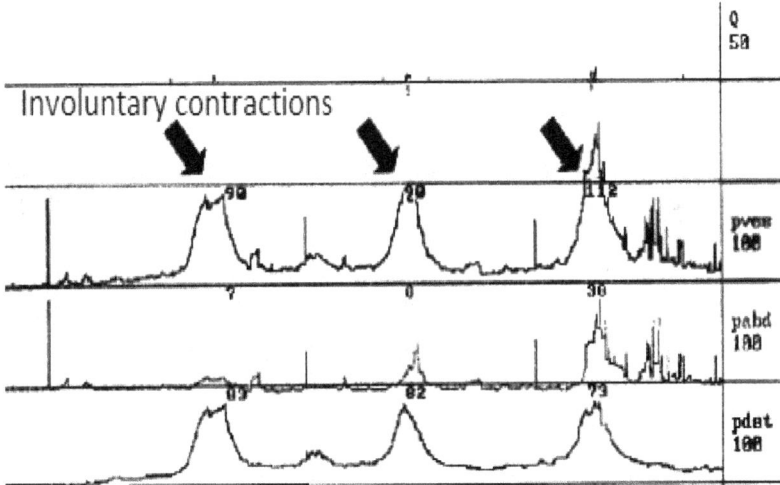

Fig. 24. Urodynamic detrusor over activity.

Since the first voiding sensation to the end of a normal filling phase (full bladder sensation), the patient is asked to increase the abdominal pressure in a way that would normally produce stress incontinence (cough, etc.). If urine leakage is registered with these manoeuvres, urodynamic stress incontinence is diagnosed (Fig. 25).

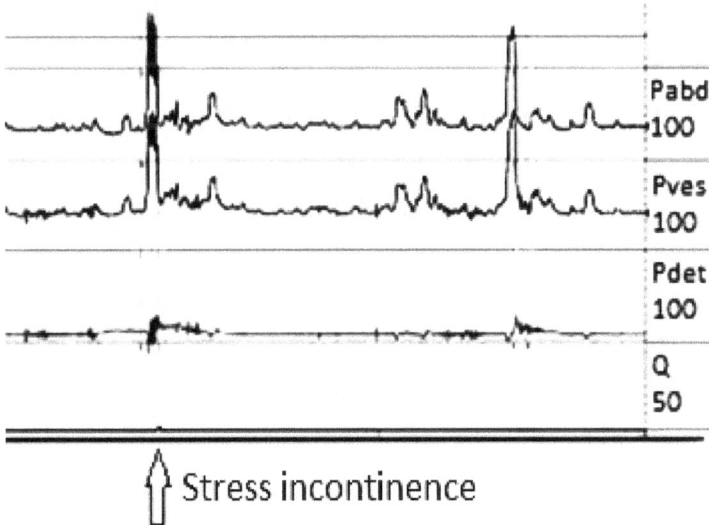

Fig. 25. Urodynamic stress incontinence.

Consider repeating the study, performing ambulatory urodynamics (portable equipment) or video-urodynamics if the diagnosis is not clear after a conventional study.

Other studies may be indicated according to clinical findings, such as CT scanning or MRI (extra-urethral incontinence, fistulae, etc.).

With all this information a precise or very accurate diagnosis of UI can be obtained, as well as the type and the cause or causes producing it, so a rational treatment plan can be organised.

CONCLUSION.

This table summarises the **clinical** diagnosis:

	Urge UI	Stress UI	Mixed UI
Sudden desire to void	+	-	+
8 or > voids per day	+	-	+
Leak at cough, sneeze	-	+	+
Can hold till WC	-	+	-
Voids at night	+	-	+

Fig. 26. Table with guidance towards clinical diagnosis.

ADDITIONAL READING.

1. Initial Assessment of Urinary and Faecal Incontinence in Adult Male and Female Patients. Staskin D, Kelleher C, Bosch R, Coyne K, Cotterill N, Emmanuel A, Yoshida M, Kopp Z. In: Incontinence. Abrams P, Cardozo L, Khoury S, Wein A. Eds. Health Publication Ltd. France. 2009.
2. Incontinencia Urinaria. Castro Díaz D, González R. Pulso Ediciones. DL: B-854-1993.

CHAPTER 3. URODYNAMIC STUDIES.

Mintegui D and Clavijo J.

The main objective of UDS is to reproduce the patient's symptoms and relate them to the study's findings, so the clinical question that led to the study can be answered. The success of the study depends on a meticulous setup of the equipment and strict quality control through each one of the procedures.

Standardization and good practice for doing the study and for quality control in the various UDS follow the nomenclature and advice of the ICS.

MINIMAL TECHNICAL REQUIREMENTS OF THE EQUIPMENT.

Precision of ± 1 cm H2O for pressures and ± 5% of the complete scale for volume. Recording ranges have to be 0-250 cm H2O for pressures, 0-50 ml/s for flow and 0-1000 ml for volume. During recording and analysis minimum pressure scale must be 50 cm H2O by cm for pressures, 10 ml/s by cm for flow and 1 min/cm or 5 s/mm during filling and 2 s/mm during voiding for time scale.

Calibration of equipment must be done regularly, especially if transducers are changed and it must not be confused with "zero setting". Calibration of flowmeters is done by pouring a precise volume at a known flow rate. This is achieved by special constant flow bottles. It's advisable to check the infusion pump with the filling lines connected, checking the time the pump takes to deliver a pre-determined volume. Pressure transducers can be checked by raising the connexion lines over the reference line a pre-determined distance in cm, which has to be reflected in the reading.

When software is used to analyse the information obtained, the source of the software has to be referenced, and whether it has been validated.

FLOW RATE.

This is a non-invasive measurement of urinary flow during the voiding phase. It's influenced by 3 variables: Pdet, urethral calibre and urethral closure system relaxation. Flow rate is the volume of urine (ml) voided per time unit (s). It's measured in ml/s. To be reliable, it needs to be obtained in privacy, and with a normal bladder fullness sensation and a minimal voiding volume of 150 ml. The values recorded are: voided volume, maximum flow rate (Qmax), time to Qmax, and pattern of the curve (Fig. 27). It always has to be recorded together with the corresponding post micturition residual volume (PVR or PMR).

Qmax is the highest reading during micturition. It's very well related with the presence of obstruction. Qmax values below 10-12 ml/s are related with a high likelihood of infra-vesical obstruction. Rates of 12-15 are less likely, and above 15 ml/s the possibility of obstruction is very low. However, always keep in mind that a normal flow can be achieved in an obstructed system by increasing Pves. The opposite can also happen, and there can be a low flow (<10 ml/s) without obstruction due to low Pves, such as in detrusor failure (with low Pdet). Therefore for an unequivocal diagnosis of obstruction, a more invasive pressure/flow study is needed.

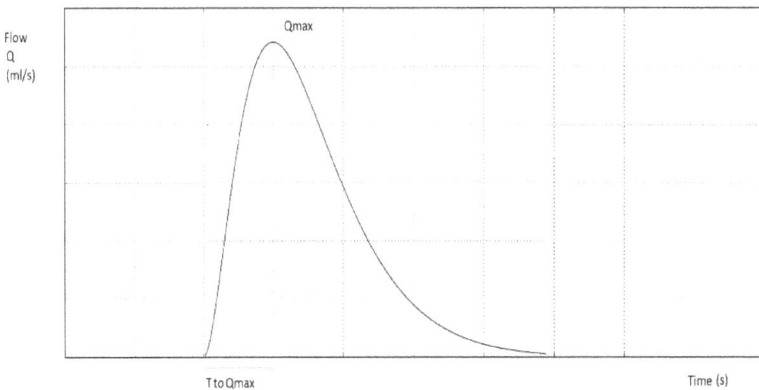

Fig. 27. Analysis of flow rate.

The technical report from the ICS recommends these standards for flowmeters: range between 0-50 ml/s for flow, 0-1000 for volume and ± 5% accuracy. Therefore it is unnecessary to report anything beyond 1 ml/s (no decimals). As most flowmeters measure mass (weight on rotating disc), the density of urine has to be considered. As an example, highly concentrated urine can raise artificially the flow rate registered up to 3%, and contrast media (used in video UDS) up to 10%.

To facilitate recognition of flow patterns, the flow trace should be standard. One millimetre of paper should equal 1 second in the horizontal axis (X), and 1 ml/s in the vertical axis (Y).

The ICS advises to **smooth the curve by hand**, drawing a continuous line, so that every 2 seconds there are no sharp changes, and only then calculate the Qmax (Fig. 28).

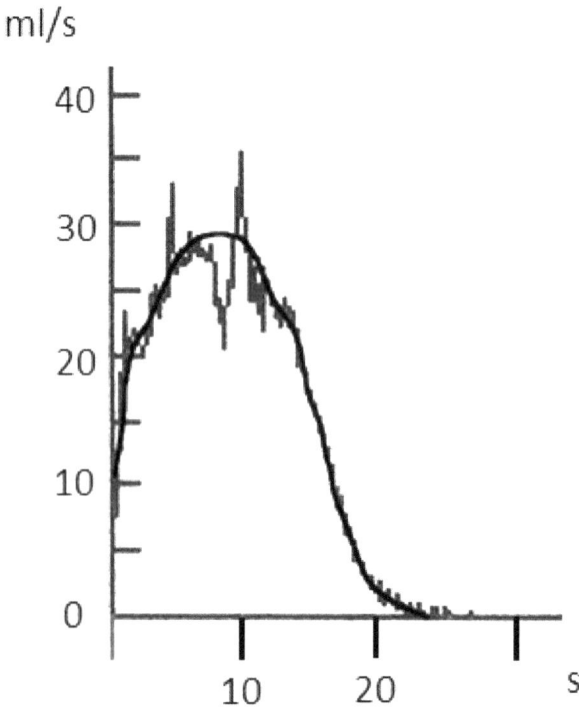

Fig. 28. Corrected Qmax. Flow rate from a rotating disc. Uncorrected Qmax is 36 ml/s, Voided volume (Vvol) is 390 ml, without PVR. After corrected, smoothed curve, the Qmax is just below 30 ml/s.

Qmax should be rounded to the closest whole number (e.g. 10.25 ml/s is 10 ml/s) and Vvol to the closest 10 ml (e.g. Vvol 342 ml is 340 ml).

The best way to register Qmax is with the Vvol and PVR using this format:
Qmax (ml/s) / Vvol (ml) / PVR (ml). Use a line if any of the values are missing (e.g. 10 ml/s / 340 ml /---).

Flowmetry can produce several **flow patterns**:
- Normal (bell shaped, with a quick rise looking like a Poisson distribution)
- Slow (prolonged voiding time)

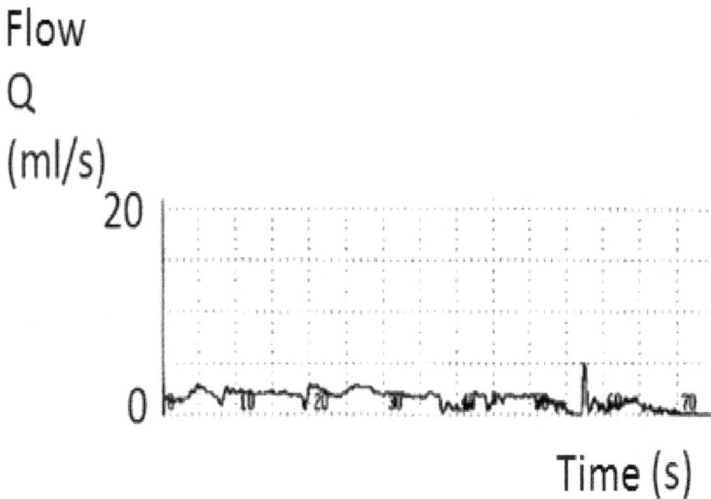

Fig. 29. Reduced and slow flow.

- intermittent (irregular spikes)

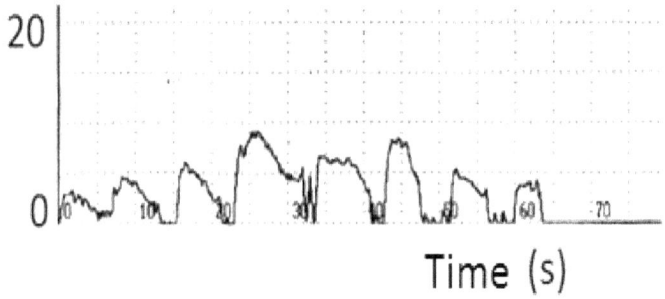

Fig. 30. Intermittent flow.

- flat or plateau (reduced Qmax with prolonged time)

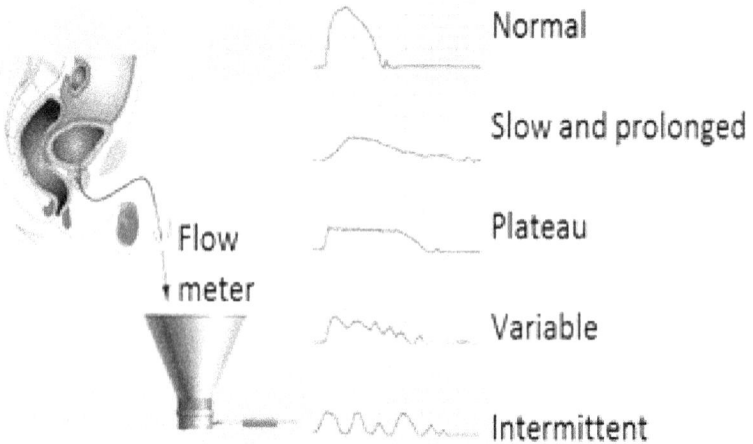

Fig. 31. Normal and abnormal flow patterns.

FILLING CYSTOMETRY.

It's the simultaneous recording of Pves and Pabd during a bladder filling (usually with normal saline).
Three pressures are recorded:
- Pves (bladder transducer): total pressure within the bladder.
- Pabd (rectal transducer, more rarely vaginal or in a colostomy): pressure around the bladder.
- Pdet or subtraction pressure: it is calculated by subtracting Pabd to Pves (Pdet = Pves − Pabd).

To measure Pves and fill the bladder a standard two lumen catheter is usually used. This should be as thin as possible. The inner lumen should allow for an adequate pressure registry and adequate infusion flow. The main advantage of a dual lumen catheter (versus two single catheters) is that the filling/voiding cycle can be repeated without the need to replace a filling catheter. A 6 Fr double lumen catheter (the smallest standard) can limit infusion flow to 20-30 ml/min. This in turn may create a conflict with the infusion pump reading. On the other hand, the use of 2 single lumen catheters, one for filling and one for recording Pves, is less convenient. The withdrawal of the filling catheter before voiding is an advantage, leaving only a thin catheter in the urethra. However, this advantage is outweighed by the need to re-catheterise the patient, if another filling cycle is needed.

Information from the cystometry:
- First voiding sensation   (150-200 ml)
- Maximum bladder capacity (450-500 ml)

To measure Pabd use a balloon rectal catheter. In females this can also be placed in the upper part of the vagina with similar results. The balloon should hold a small volume of fluid at the tip of the catheter to avoid blockage by faeces. Additionally as the rectum and vagina are not filled with fluid, the balloon prevents recording artefacts produced by contact of the tip of the catheter and the wall of the organ. The balloon works best when it's filled to 20% of its capacity. A very common error in Pabd recording is the use of an over distended balloon, which will yield an elevated false reading. This can be prevented by creating a puncture or orifice in the balloon. There are some balloon catheters that come with a factory made hole (communication).

Standards for reference height and zeroing.
The ICS recommends the use of normal saline filled lines for measurement of pressures connected to external pressure transducers. This facilitates zeroing and placement at the reference level. This recommendation needs to be followed closely as it's the only way to compare recordings from different patients and different clinics in a meaningful way.

Zero pressure is atmospheric pressure. When the transducer is directly open to ambient pressure only, the "zeroing" has to be done with the equipment calibration system. **Reference height or level is the superior part of the symphysis pubis.** This is the level at which the transducers have to be placed before zeroing so all pressures will have the same hydrostatic component. This is a real and relevant range and one of the critical quality control points. Some readings are made on Pves, like Valsalva leak point pressure (VLPP), which is sensitive to reference level (unlike Pdet measurements).

Any changes in patient position has to be compensated for, by repositioning the transducers at the symphysis level, otherwise the readings will be incorrect (Fig. 32). This is frequently the case when the patient stands up during the study.

External pressure transducers measure pressure according to their relative position to the bladder, regardless of the position of the tip of the catheter. As an example, if placed at the level of the symphysis it measures 15 cm H2O, by raising it 9 cm; it will read 6 cm H2O.

Quality control of pressures and basic corrections.
Before starting a UDS it's important to check carefully the pressure signals and correct any problems. The first objective is to avoid artefacts and the second is to correct them should they appear.

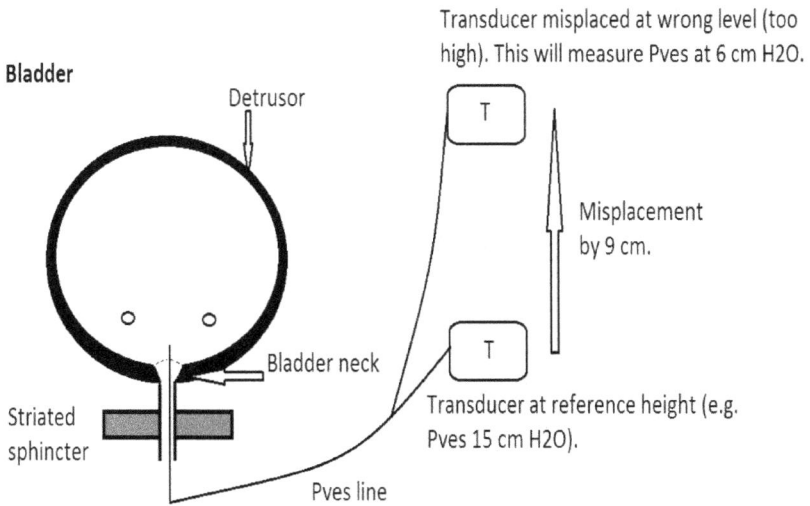

Fig. 32. Effect of reference height of the transducer.

If readings are adequate at the beginning they tend to remain so during the course of the study. Checklist:

1. initial Pabd and Pves ranges are normal: supine 5-20 cm H2O, sitting 15-40 cm H2O, and standing 30-50 cm H2O.

Usual ranges of Pabd and Pves at rest:

Position	P pressure (cm H2O)
Supine	5 – 20
Sitting	15 – 40
Standing	30 – 50

2. Correct initial alterations in Pdet: usually Pabd and Pves are similar, so initial Pdet is zero, or close to zero. Initial Pdet are 0 to 6 cm H2O in 80% of readings, rarely reaching 10 cm H2O. However, initial Pdet can be acceptable from -5 to 15 cm H2O.

Problems:

a. High Pdet:

- Pabd can be too low due to the rectal line or its connections being blocked or kinked. There can also be air bubbles inside or a fluid leak. The systems needs to be flushed, any kinks straightened and leaks ruled out.

- Pves can be too high if the tip of the catheter has moved down to the urethra or the catheter or connections are kinked. Rule out kinks and reposition if necessary.

b. Negative Pdet:
- Pabd too high due to the catheter displaced or contacting the rectal wall or the catheter or connections are kinked. Check position and rule out bending. The rectal balloon can be over distended, so it has to be drained to 20% of its capacity.
- Pves too low due to the line or connections blocked or bent; there are air bubbles in the system or there is a fluid leak. The system has to be flushed and bending and fluid leaks excluded. Air is compressible, so bubbles act as pressure cushioning, lowering the readings.

3. Confirm that the readings from Pabd and Pves are live. They will have small variations caused by breathing or talking, similar in both tracings, and that should not affect Pdet.

4. After checking that resting pressures are within a normal range, you have to **check pressure transmission. If there are any buffers they have to be detected and corrected.** This is done by asking the patient to cough; both Pabd and Pves must rise and fall briefly and equally, without a significant change in Pdet. A small up and down (biphasic) symmetric change in Pdet is also considered normal (due to delay in registry from the transducers). Any ascent or descent in Pdet is likely to be a cushioning or buffering in the recording or Pabd or Pves respectively (Fig. 33).

Pressure transmission and damping throughout the registry has to be checked by asking the patient to cough. This has to be performed at the beginning and end of the filling phase, every minute during the filling process, before and after any major event, like position changes and leakage and voiding, since all these events can dislodge the catheters. Usually damping happens in the line that responds less to cough; this has to be corrected as soon as detected by flushing the line and ruling out kinks.

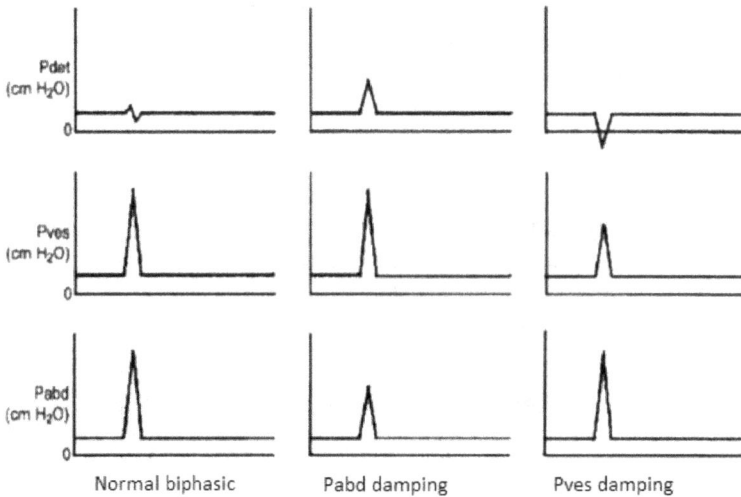

Fig. 33. Pressures transmission. Left: good transmission and subtraction without damping. Centre: damping of Pabd. Right: damping of Pves.

5. Sudden pressure changes suggest that either the rectal or bladder catheter has been displaced. Either can come out completely with a complete and dramatic pressure drop or they can move to a higher pressure area (like the urethra or anal canal). This needs repositioning or changing if they fell in a non-sterile area.

Cystometry is indicated when detrusor over activity is suspected and in mixed UI. It's also necessary in patients that don't respond to standard non-invasive treatment or when an invasive treatment is planned. It's always necessary in patients with incontinence and neurological disease as well as those who had previous pelvic operations.

During the study it is recommended to record subjective symptoms such as: urgency, pain, voiding sensations, unusual symptoms (perspiration, dizziness, etc.). Objective signs: maximum bladder capacity (MBC), volumes at which different symptoms appear, presence or absence of involuntary contractions (IDC), volume at first IDC, incontinence with cough, Valsalva manoeuvre, end filling Pdet and Pves.

Bladder compliance (C) or distensibility is the change in Pves for a change in volume (C= dV/dPves). It is expressed in ml/cmH2O. Normal values are above 20 ml/cm H2O.

During the filling phase there should be no detrusor contractions. Any rise in Pdet either spontaneous or secondary to a trigger manoeuvre (cough, change in position, hearing running water, wet hands, and cold feet) is an involuntary detrusor contraction (IDC). Bladder over activity (OAB) or hyperactivity is the situation when the bladder contracts during filling (IDCs). There are two types of OAB:

- Bladder hyper-reflexia: when there is objective evidence of a neurological disease (SCI, CVA, demyelinising disease, etc.). The IDCs during filling are secondary to neurological control lesions.
- Idiopathic OAB: IDCs are not related to neurologic damage. They may be associated to obstruction, irritation or produced by unknown mechanisms.

Leak point pressures (LPP).
LPP it's Pves at the point of incontinence at a certain filling volume. Types of LPP:
1. Detrusor leak point pressure (DLPP): it's Pves during leak triggered by an IDC. It is linked to the resistance of the urethral closure system to the rise in Pves due to a detrusor contraction. It is a prognostic factor for upper urinary tract damage if DLPP is higher than 40 cm H2O.
2. Valsalva leak point pressure (VLPP): it's Pves during leak triggered by a stress manoeuvre. Useful in SUI. VLPPs under 60 cm H2O are suggestive of a degree of intrinsic sphincter deficiency (ISD), which is certain with VLPPs under 30 cm H2O.

Pressure-flow study (P/Q).
It's the simultaneous measurement of Pves and flow rate during voiding. This study is the objective assessment of whether there is an infravesical obstruction or not. It identifies poor flows secondary to detrusor failure. It assesses flow and the Pves used to produce it. Under normal circumstances it will identify patients with low Qmax secondary to obstruction from those secondary to impaired detrusor contraction. It can also identify patients with

obstruction with high pressures and relatively normal or indeterminate flow. The diagnoses that can be made are:

a) Infravesical obstruction: diagnosed with low flow in the presence of a detrusor contraction of sufficient pressure, duration and speed. In a simple way is Qmax < 15 ml/s with Pdet > 40 cm H2O.

b) Underactive detrusor: a low flow is suspicious but not diagnostic of obstruction. Underactive detrusor is low Qmax with Pdet < 40 cm H2O and usually under 20 cm H2O. This poor detrusor contraction can be a consequence of a neurological problem or detrusor muscle damage, like in over-distention, ageing, fibrosis, scars, and diverticula.

Normally there is no delay between Pves rise and the flow to start. Both tracings should be synchronized. As flow is registered outside the urethra, the registry shows a delay. This delay increases with the distance between the bladder neck and the flowmeter. It is also increased by the mechanical delay of the meter. When P/Q studies are analysed a delay of 0.5 – 2 seconds has to be considered, this can be relevant if there are fast changes in pressure or flow.

There is another delay between urethral closure and the end of the recording, which can be longer, particularly in benign prostatic obstruction. Therefore pressures should be described as at initial flow and end of flow rather than opening or closing.

Additional considerations.
During filling cystometry always register:
1. Infusion speed: it is considered physiological if it's lower than the patients weight divided by 4 (in kg), expressed in ml/min. Any speed higher is not physiological (and it's used as a trigger for IDCs).

2. Temperature of infusion fluid (or gas), which is usually normal saline (at room or body temperature). Anything colder than body temperature is also a trigger for IDCs. It's contraindicated to infuse anything at above body temperature (36 °C).

3. Position of the patient: supine, sitting, standing.

4. Other manoeuvres to trigger IDCs: position changes, wet hands, cough, Valsalva manoeuvre, listening to running water, sensation of cold, etc.

ELECTROMYOGRAM (EMG).

It's the registry of the electrical activity originated by striated muscles cells membrane depolarization when stimulated by a nerve. The electrodes are located to receive the activity of the levator ani. Besides diagnosing a neurological lesion, it can also identify a functional obstruction by detrusor-sphincter dyssynergia. Detrusor-sphincter dyssynergia is the increase in EMG activity of the striated sphincter muscle during detrusor contraction. This is a physio-pathological situation that can be neurogenic (like in SCI) or a learned behaviour (like in Fowler's or Hinman's syndromes). There are two types of dyssynergia: detrusor-bladder neck (which requires a radiological diagnosis, and has no EMG alterations) and detrusor-striated sphincter dyssynergia (Fig. 35).

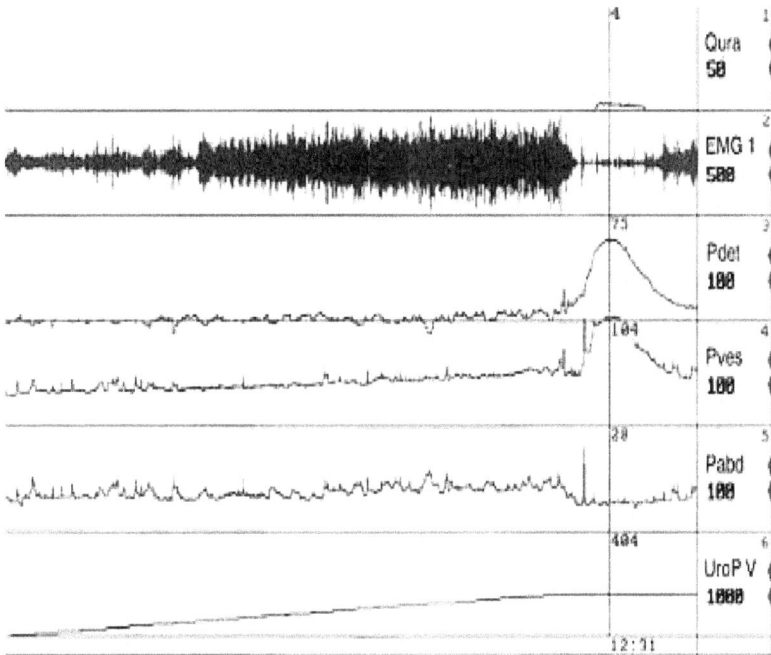

Fig. 34. UDS shows non-neurogenic obstruction (high pressures + low flow) with a normal EMG.

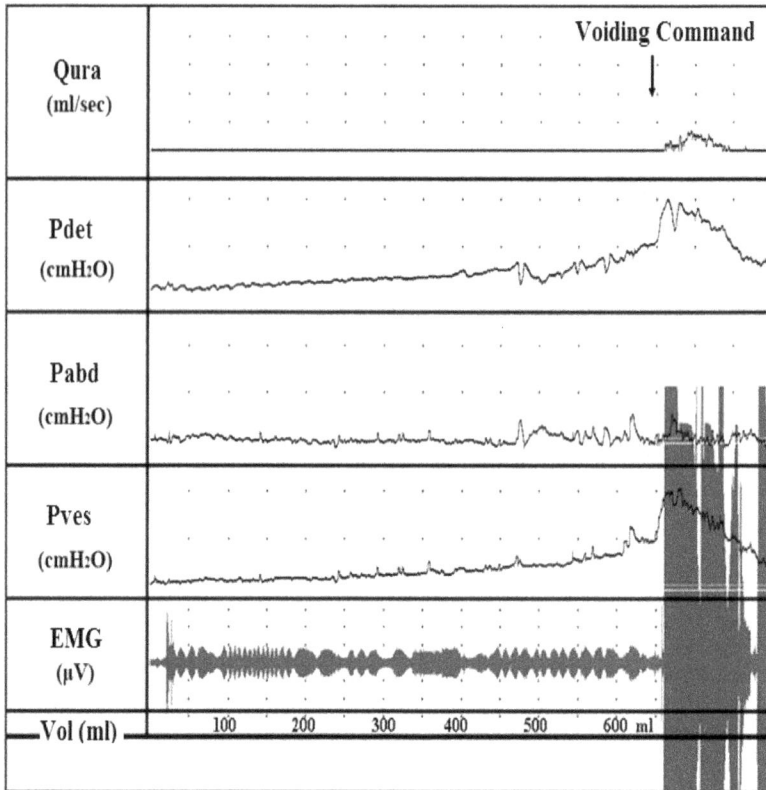

Fig. 35. UDS shows obstruction (high pressures + low flow) with a
dyssynergic EMG (increased EMG activity during voiding and
detrusor contraction).[ix]

VIDEOURODYNAMICS.

It's the simultaneous recording of a complete UDS and a video of radioscopic images of the lower urinary tract. The radioscopic images are obtained using saline or water with radiological contrast dye as the filling fluid. This shows pressure and anatomical changes at the same time (cysto-urethrogram). Video UDS are very useful in neurological patients with suspected dyssynergia, bladder neck dysfunction or functional vesico-ureteric reflux (VUR). (Fig. 36).

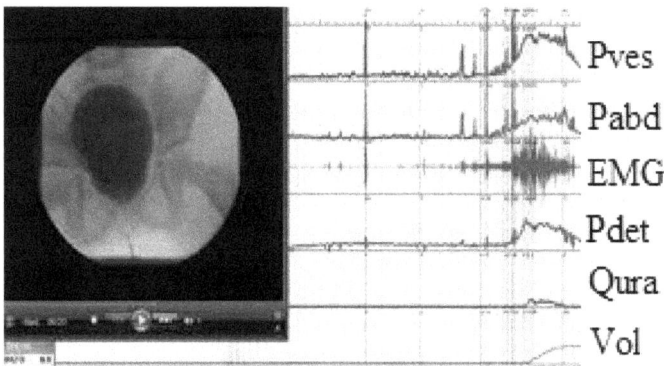

Fig. 36. Video UDS[x].

CONCLUSION.

Invasive UDS should only be performed with a precise indication, having made a clinical question that needs to be answered by the study. Main recommendations include:

- A good UDS has to be done in interaction with the patient, asking whether the symptoms were reproduced during the study.
- There must be a careful and continuous observation of the data as they are obtained and a continuous evaluation of their mutual correlations.
- Artefacts are to be avoided, and corrected immediately if they happen, as it's difficult or impossible to do so retrospectively.
- If a patient has a prolapse, bladder and urethral function should be assessed after its correction.

ADDITIONAL READING.

1. Estandarización y control de calidad en los estudios urodinámicos. Valdevenito JP. Rev Hosp Clín Univ Chile. 2012; 23: 123 – 33.
2. The standardisation of terminology in lower urinary tract function. Abrams P, Cardozo L, Fall M, Griffiths D, Rosier P, Ulmsten U et al. Neurourol Urodyn 2002; 21: 67-78.
3. Good urodynamic practices: uroflowmetry, filling cystometry, and pressure-flow studies. Schäfer W, Abrams P, Liao L, Mattiasson A, Pesce F, Spangberg A et al. Neurourol Urodyn 2002; 21:261-74.
4. Basic principles of urodynamic measurements. Drinnan M, Griffiths C, Hosker G. Regional Medical Physics Department. Freeman Hospital, Newcastle Upon Tyne, United Kingdom 2004.
5. Voiding dysfunction and urodynamic abnormalities in elderly patients. Gomes Cristiano M., Arap S, Trigo-Rocha F E. Rev. Hosp. Clin. 2004; 59(4): 206-215.
6. Urodynamics made easy. Chapple C, MacDiarmid SA, Patel A. Third edition. Edinburgh: Churchill Livingstone, 2009.

CHAPTER 4. TREATMENT OF URINARY INCONTINENCE.

Craviotto F, Chiba W, Dieppa V, Varela M and Clavijo J.

Treatment of UI can be medical, surgical or palliative with collection devices or a combination of these. The choice of treatment will depend of many factors, especially the prognosis of underlying conditions in neurological patients. Physical and mental capacity, motivation and carers support all have to be given serious consideration.

The first step to try to correct incontinence is using dietary and hygienic measures with behaviour modification and pelvic muscles physiotherapy. This requires timely patient education towards self-help in a way that can be understood and implemented.

The second additional rung is medication.

A third rung includes treatment options that are considered and implemented by a coordinated multidisciplinary team: supervised behaviour modification, biofeedback, supervised pelvic muscles physiotherapy, functional peripheral electrical stimulation and neuromodulation, and surgical interventions.

It's necessary to know the correct use of medications and palliative alternatives as well as the surgical options. Do not perform invasive UDS before non-surgical management.

LIFESTYLE MEASURES.

Bladder re-training: for OAB, UUI and MUI. Offer for 4-6 weeks minimum as first line option. This includes:

- Diet and hydration: patients with incontinence benefit from a close control of the fluid they consume to produce an adequate volume of urine (diuresis). An excessive diuresis worsens incontinence. For this reason, also avoid food and drinks with a diuretic effect, like alcohol, tea, coffee and other caffeinated drinks. **Patients with a BMI over 30 improve their continence by weight reduction.**
- Timing: people with UI improve by organising when they drink fluids. It's better to drink more in the morning and reducing the volume in the afternoon and evening.
- Adequate voiding frequency: this allows for a better control of incontinent episodes should they happen. Keeping the bladder with a lower volume helps with protection measures and avoids stimuli from an overstretched bladder. In OAB and UUI always leave home with an empty bladder and do not overdrink whilst out, especially if toilet facilities are scarce or inadequate. In patients with cognitive impairment, organize prompted voiding with a schedule.
- Voiding diaries: they are of great help as a feedback tool. The patient becomes aware of voiding habits as well as fluid/food consumption. They register volume passed and intake, as well as the time all events happen, including urgency, incontinence and protection used. They have to be filled before the 1st appointment (or immediately afterwards) and after each intervention to assess the results (together with the other assessment forms). There are several mobile phone applications available to use.
- Adequate body and perineal hygiene training and house/work adaptation in patients that require it.
- It's generally advisable to increase dietary fibre to **avoid constipation**, reduce fluid intake in the evening, avoid bladder irritants, like caffeine, alcohol and spices and **increase physical activity.**

PHARMACOLOGICAL BASIS OF TREATMENT.

There are several medications that act on the bladder and urethra that can be used to improve continence. Continence and voiding are mainly controlled by the autonomous nervous system. The filling phase relies on the adrenergic activity that closes the bladder neck (alpha receptors) and that relaxes the detrusor (beta receptors). Voiding depends on the cholinergic activity that produces contraction of the detrusor and the suppression of the adrenergic activity on the bladder neck.

There are several groups of medications that can be useful in the treatment of incontinence:
- Medications that reduce detrusor contractility like anticholinergics and beta adrenergic agonists.
- Medications that increase urethral resistance like alpha adrenergic agonists.
- Medications that improve urethral and bladder tissue quality, and response to medication. Particularly local vaginal oestrogens that improve vaginal trophism and the number of receptors in the area.

Unlike other organs (like the heart) where there are medications that are organ-specific and produce their effect almost exclusively in the target organ, with very few side effects; there are no medications with exclusive action at the bladder or urethra. This means that the available medications for continence also act on other organs and systems and produce side effects that can be **mild to severe**. This is so relevant that side effects are responsible for a 50% abandonment rate in continence medications in the first year of use.

MEDICATION	DOSIS	EFFECTS
Oxybutynin	5-10 mg TDS p.o.	Detrusor relaxation, local anaesthetic
Tolterodine	2 mg BID	Detrusor relaxation
Solifenacin	5-10 mg OD	Detrusor relaxation
Fesoterodine	4-8 mg OD	Detrusor relaxation
Trospium chloride	20-30 mg BID	Detrusor relaxation
Flavoxate	200 mg QDS	Detrusor relaxation
Imipramine	25 mg TDS	Detrusor relaxation, bladder neck closure, increase in striated sphincter tone
Duloxetine	80 mg OD	Bladder neck closure, increase in striated sphincter tone
Desmopressin	0.2-0.4 mg OD	Antidiuretic
Mirabegron	25-50 mg OD	Detrusor relaxation
Propantheline bromide	15 mg QDS	Detrusor relaxation

Fig. 37. Some medications used in incontinence with their mechanism of action and usual adult dose.

URGE URINARY INCONTINENCE.

The objective of bladder over activity treatment is to obtain a bladder that can distend during the filling phase and that can accommodate a good volume of urine. This goal is occasionally obtainable, but in many patients we can only get a reduction in frequency and a reduction in the number of incontinent episodes (which has the greater impact in quality of life). Before treating an OAB we need to know its origin, rule out neurological disease, rule out bladder diseases like cancer, stones, infection and inflammations; and also anal, rectal and gynaecological conditions that can produce OAB and need a specific treatment.

Once a correct diagnosis is reached and other pathology ruled out, we can consider the management alternatives that include: lifestyle interventions, pharmacological treatment, bladder re-training, pelvic muscles exercises (PME). The last two will rely on behavioural modification, physiotherapy, biofeedback, electrical stimulation and neuromodulation. Finally there are surgical options. Palliative measures like external penile collectors, collecting bags, catheters and absorbent products can be used in non-responders, before a definitive treatment, or those that due to age, comorbidities or poor performance status are not suitable for invasive treatments. These strategies and devices can keep the patient dry, avoid contact of the skin with urine and ensuing skin lesions; and allow the patient to be **socially integrated**.

The treatment plan should follow some treatment rungs that go from less to more invasive interventions, and it always needs to be tailored to the **patient's needs and choice**.

Treatment rungs.
- Lifestyle interventions.
- Behavioural modification techniques. Timed voiding.
- Physiotherapy. PME.
- Medication.
- Biofeedback.
- Electro-stimulation.
- Neuromodulation:
  - Peripheral. Tibial nerve stimulation (PTNS).

o Central (implantable electrodes). Sacral root stimulation.
- Surgery. Botulinum toxin A injection. Bladder augmentation. External urinary diversion.
- Palliative treatments (at any level and according to patient's comorbidities and preferences).

PME physiotherapy.
This treatment is a series of techniques oriented to develop and strengthen the muscles of the pelvis and to modify the voiding habits of the patient to improve their self-control over the voiding-filling cycle. This includes supervised PME (also called Kegel) at least for 3 months (Fig. 38).

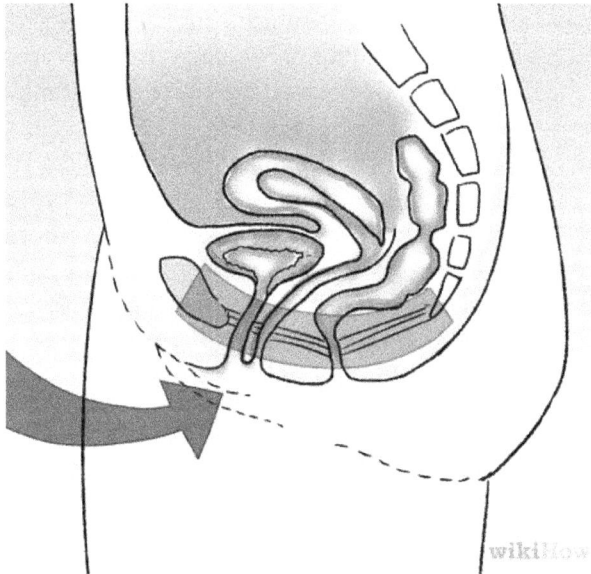

Fig. 38. PME.

Medication.
Anticholinergics are the most frequently used medications for the treatment of detrusor over activity. Since bladder contraction is mediated by acetylcholine, the blockage of post-ganglionic cholinergic receptors in the detrusor produces relaxation. Muscarinic receptors are widely distributed in many organs, which explain the side effects including dry mouth, constipation, and blurred vision. They are contraindicated in close angle

glaucoma, megacolon, myasthenia gravis and untreated tachycardia. They can produce an increase in PMR particularly if there is an associated outflow obstruction, especially in men. The same applies for patients with detrusor hyperactivity with impaired contractility (DHIC), frequently seen in the elderly. Except for Trospium, which does not cross the blood-brain barrier, they're contraindicated in patients with cognitive impairment.

Anticholinergics reduce detrusor contractility, increase bladder capacity and consequently reduce frequency and episodes of urgency and UUI. Symptoms improvement is not immediate, as voiding habits modification is a gradual process. Therefore clinical response has to be assessed after a period of 3-6 weeks. In neurogenic patients with hyper-reflexia and dyssynergia there are high intravesical pressures during voiding. This can irreversibly damage the upper urinary tract leading to end stage renal failure.

In patients at high risk of renal damage (Pves > 40 cm H2O), the use of anticholinergics is necessary (or an alternative detrusor relaxation treatment) combined with intermittent catheterisation to empty the bladder. No anticholinergic has been consistently proven better than others, but side effect profiles may vary and a patient may do better with a particular medication than with the rest. As with other medication groups, it may be necessary for patients to try several of them before finding the one with the best efficacy/side effect profile for them.

Patients' assessment of anticholinergics' benefits show:
- 15% no improvement
- 35% mild improvement
- 45% significant improvement

Mirabegron is a beta agonist, which has been proven effective and better tolerated than anticholinergics. It needs to be used with caution in patients with dysrhythmias.

Neuromodulation.
Peripheral neuromodulation is tibial nerve stimulation (**PTNS**). (Fig. 39). An electrical stimulus is applied to the tibial nerve close

to the ankle. This is done with a needle and patch electrode set. These afferent stimuli arrive to the spinal centres and produce an inhibitory response on detrusor contraction (efferent loop). It is given in 1 to 3 weekly sessions for 4 to 12 weeks (12 session induction). If there is a significant improvement, the patient may need 2 to 4 monthly maintenance sessions. Each session takes 20 to 40 minutes.

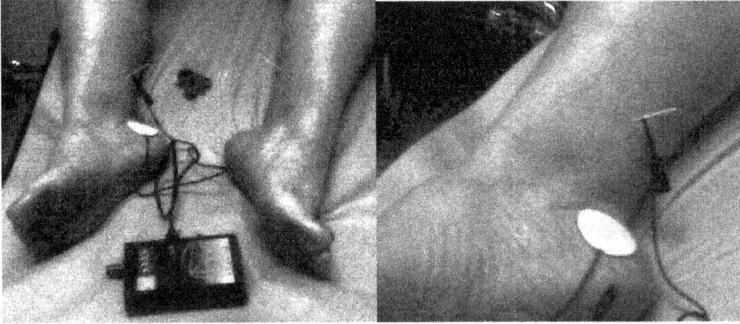

Fig. 39. Afferent nerve stimulation. PTNS.

Central neuromodulation is done via sacral roots stimulation. When UUI is secondary to detrusor over activity it can improve by the implantation of a permanent stimulator connected to the sacral roots to the nerves that control the bladder. (Fig. 40). Otherwise the mechanism of action is similar to PTNS.

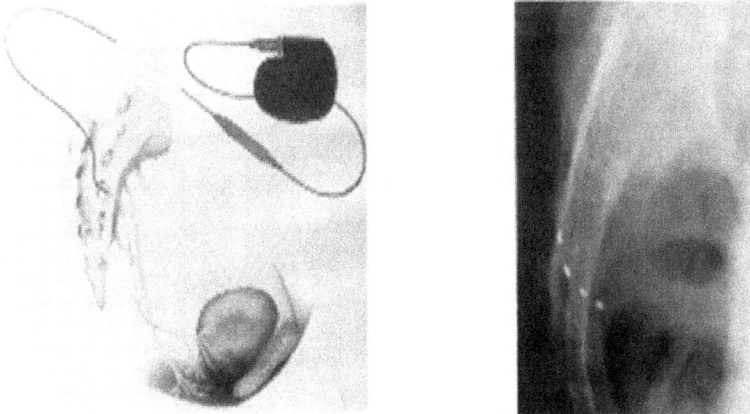

Fig. 40. Sacral roots stimulator (diagrams right and lateral x-ray left).

Intra-vesical treatments.

Botulinum toxin A can be injected in the bladder wall via a cystoscope with a special needle. This is the first line, elective treatment in patients with neurogenic bladders. Use 200 units injected in 20 to 30 points in the bladder wall. The trigone is usually spared (Fig. 41). Consider 100 units for patients who are willing to accept a lower efficacy with a lower risk of complete retention (which needs intermittent catheterisation for the duration of the Botulinum toxin's effect). These tend to be patients with idiopathic OAB and UUI. The injections need to be repeated every 6 to 12 months, when symptoms re-appear.

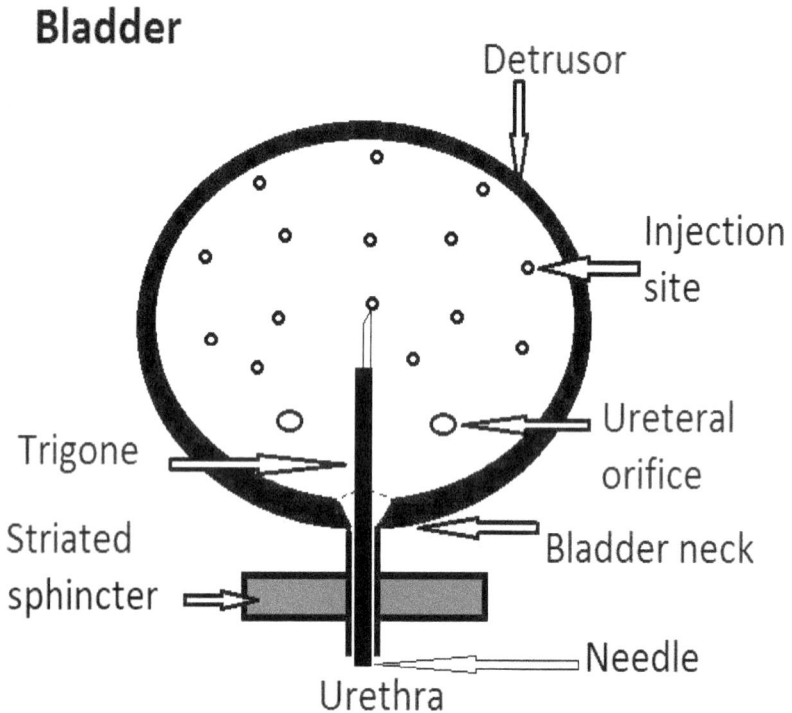

Fig. 41. Bladder botulinum toxin injections.

Other surgical treatments.

In patients who have failed all the previous combined approaches, particularly with neurogenic detrusor over activity and incontinence, a surgical procedure can reduce bladder pressure and increase bladder capacity. This can be achieved by means of denervation (now rarely used), or bladder augmentation techniques. The most frequent augmentation technique is enterocystoplasty using a segment of ileum. This segment is detubularized and re-formed into a patch, which is applied on the bladder after a "U" shaped incision is performed on the anterior wall (clam ileocystoplasty). (Fig. 42).

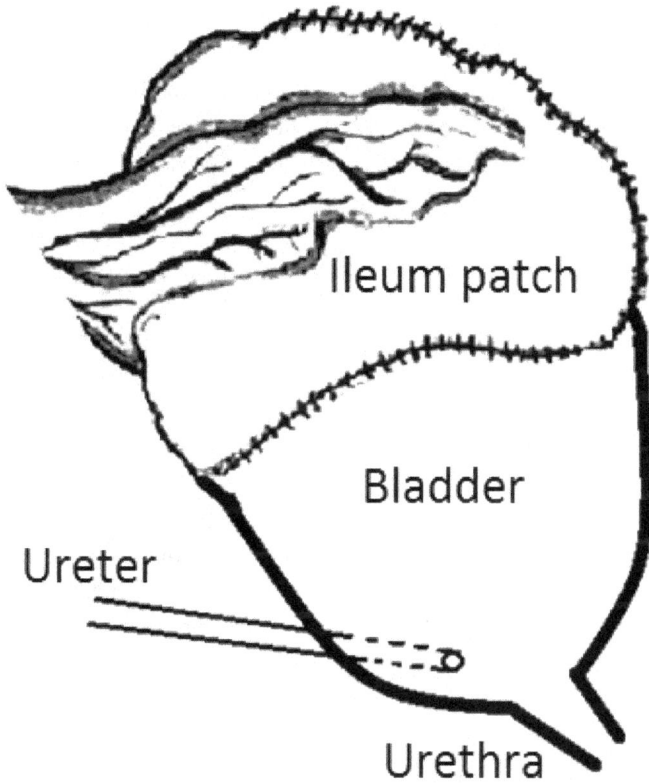

Fig. 42. Clam ileocystoplasty.

STRESS URINARY INCONTINENCE.

Unlike UUI where the most frequent management is by bladder drill and medications in SUI it's PME and surgery that offer the best solutions. Lifestyle changes and medication are usually not completely effective for most patients.

Amongst the medications used for SUI are those that increase urethral resistance and they have yielded poor results in most studies. Presently no medications are prescribed for SUI due to their side effects and meagre effectiveness. The mechanism of action is by alpha adrenergic stimulation like in: ephedrine, phenylephrine and phenylpropanolamine. Duloxetine is the most effective, and can be used as second line (instead of surgery) or in patients who are so frail that could not tolerate an operation or do not want to have one.

There are palliative options like intravaginal occlusive devices (external urethral compression) that elevate the bladder neck against the symphysis pubis and place the urethra in a higher area, where it is exposed to intra-abdominal pressure rises. There are intra-urethral occlusive devices (micro-tampons) but their use is uncommon due to their results being quite discreet.

In men SUI is usually a complication after pelvic surgery (mainly prostate). The uses of penile compression devices (like penile clamps) are not an adequate or satisfactory solution in the medium or long term. Treatment in these patients is also surgical, with some of the techniques described below or their variants.

Perineal rehabilitation.
Rehabilitation treatment is a group of techniques to develop and strengthen pelvic muscles and to modify the patient's voiding habits. This improves self-control on the storage-voiding cycle. The basic techniques include:

Physiotherapy: series of PME (like Kegel) aimed to strengthen those muscles and teach the patient how to use them correctly. In cases of prolapse these exercises will strengthen the pelvic organ's support and improve protection during abdominal strain.

It also produces reflex detrusor relaxation as a response to voluntary pelvic muscles contraction. This contraction also produces active (conscious) continence during stress manoeuvres and relocation of the bladder neck and proximal urethra in an intra-pelvic location with adequate support to improve its compression.

PME programmes include these stages:
- Information (with images, placards, drawings and models) to explain the patient the physiopathology of UI, the importance of perineal muscles being in excellent condition, and their anatomical location. The patient must understand the need for their involvement and dedication during treatment and afterwards for maintenance.
- Identification, to teach the patient to correctly contract the levator ani. Some manoeuvres are anal contraction (trying to avoid passing gas), urine flow interruption (para-physiological manoeuvre), digital vaginal assessment, and perineal observation with a mirror, palpation of the perineal fibrous centre and observation of the movement of a cotton swab or balloon catheter placed in the vagina.
- Active therapy (once the patient is capable to recognize and isolate the levator contraction, he/she must train at home). Home training includes progressive stages starting with contraction on decubitus, then sitting, squatting or standing and finally levator contraction during stress situations and other daily life activities.
- Maintenance. It's the incorporation of the PME to patient's daily life permanently. The benefits obtained by PME training disappear after 10-20 weeks of abandonment.

PME should be done at least for 6 months in series of 10 repetitions of 10 seconds each contraction, followed by 5 to 10 seconds rest, at least 3 times a day (including when waking up and going to sleep).

Biofeedback: it's used to self-monitor PME **making the contractions aware to the patient**, by visualizing or hearing it. In this way agonist and antagonist muscle groups can be identified and corrections and improvements made as needed.

<u>Electrical-stimulation</u>: it's done by direct muscle stimulation (levator ani) with anal, vaginal or perineal electrodes. It results in hypertrophy of muscle cells and improves SUI and OAB. It is advisable when the **patient is unable to obtain an adequate muscle contraction on command** (Fig. 43).

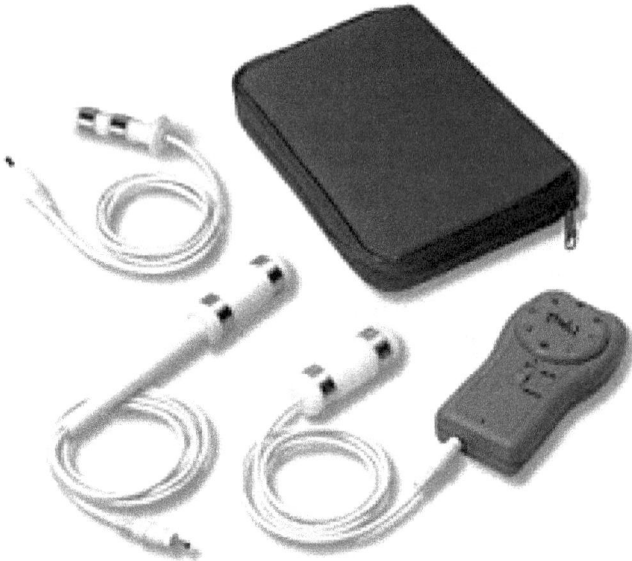

Fig. 43. Electrical stimulation devices.

Electrical stimulation and biofeedback should be entertained only in patients that are unable to willingly contract pelvic muscles in an effective way. It helps them with localisation, motivation and treatment adherence.

<u>Behaviour modification techniques</u>: it's the use of positive and negative reinforcement. This includes timed voiding (following analysis of a voiding diary), enuresis alarms (sensors that activate with dampness and generate a waking stimulus), vaginal weighted cones and relaxation techniques (yoga, meditation, acupressure and acupuncture).

Surgical treatment.
Surgery is the most effective treatment for SUI. There are several techniques for repair according to the cause of the SUI and the associated anatomical defects.

—Abdominal repair: bladder neck suspensions done open or laparoscopic. This is performed with sutures adjacent to the bladder neck and proximal urethra and fixed to bone or ligaments. They include colposuspension (Burch, etc.) and other alternatives that can be performed sub or trans-peritoneal (Fig. 44).

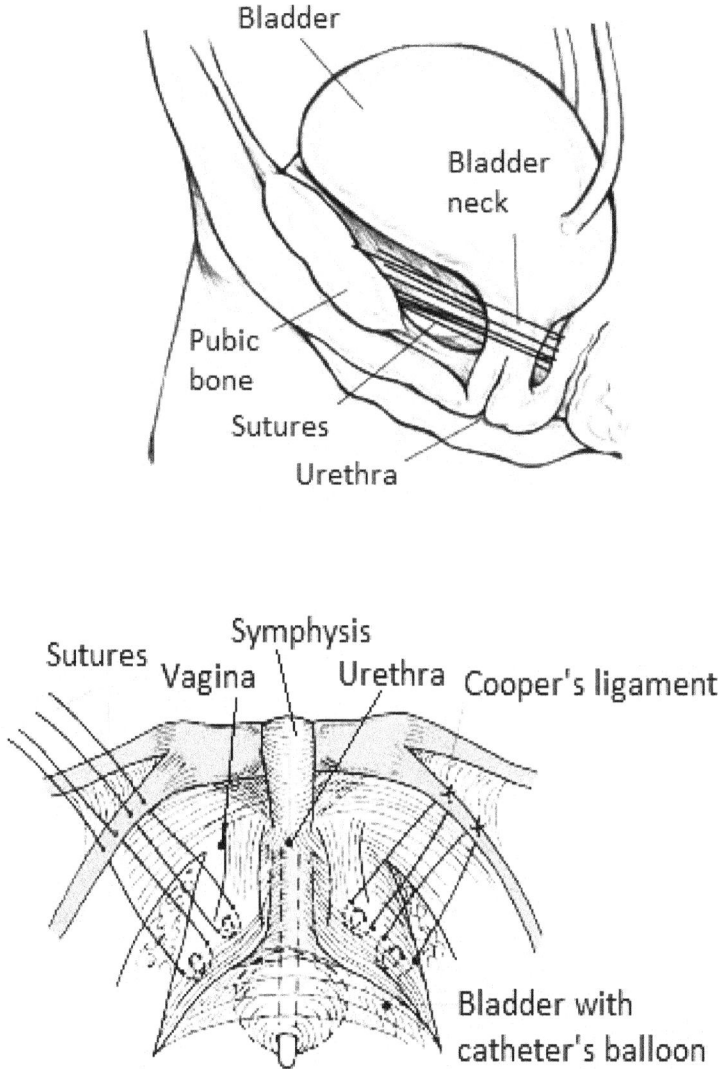

Fig. 44. Burch technique. Lateral and superior views.

— Transvaginal suspension: the urethra is held by sutures that are transferred with long needles to the suprapubic area. These techniques (Raz, Stamey, Pereyra, Gittes and their variations) are now only selectively used as they are difficult to reproduce and some may lose effectiveness with time.

— Sub-urethral slings: it's the placement of tapes or tissue patches below the urethra to provide support to the mid urethra during stress manoeuvres. They are placed without tension and without angulating the urethra. They are the most used repair for SUI and can be placed in the retro pubic area (like TVT ®) or through the obturator membrane (like TOT®). (Fig. 45).

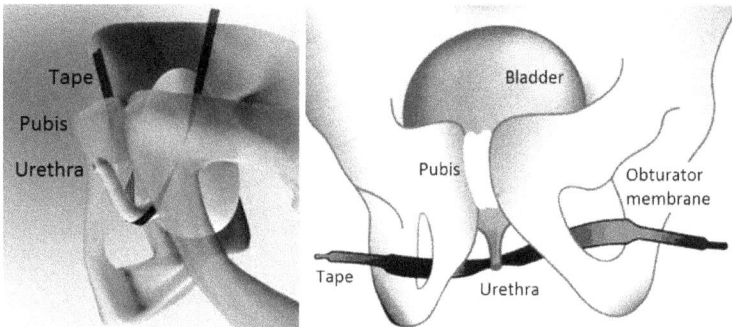

Fig. 45. Mid sub-urethral tapes. Retro pubic and trans obturator.[xi]

Sub-urethral slings are relatively easy techniques to learn and reproduce, reasonably safe, low cost and can be done under local anaesthetic as a day case and with quick recovery. Functional results amongst them are comparable, with a high cure/continence rate in the long term (> 70%). The differences amongst these operations are the anatomical approach and the sling material. Lately **there is a tendency to use autologous materials for the slings due to the long term complications of synthetic ones.** (Fig. 46).

The sling is held in place by fixation to the bone or to a ligament. Autologous materials include fascia lata, anterior rectus sheath, vaginal wall patch, etc. Synthetic materials are almost all Polypropylene meshes, with different thickness, edges, thread size and pore size. Polyethylene and Polytetrafluoroethylene slings have been abandoned due to an even higher complication rate.

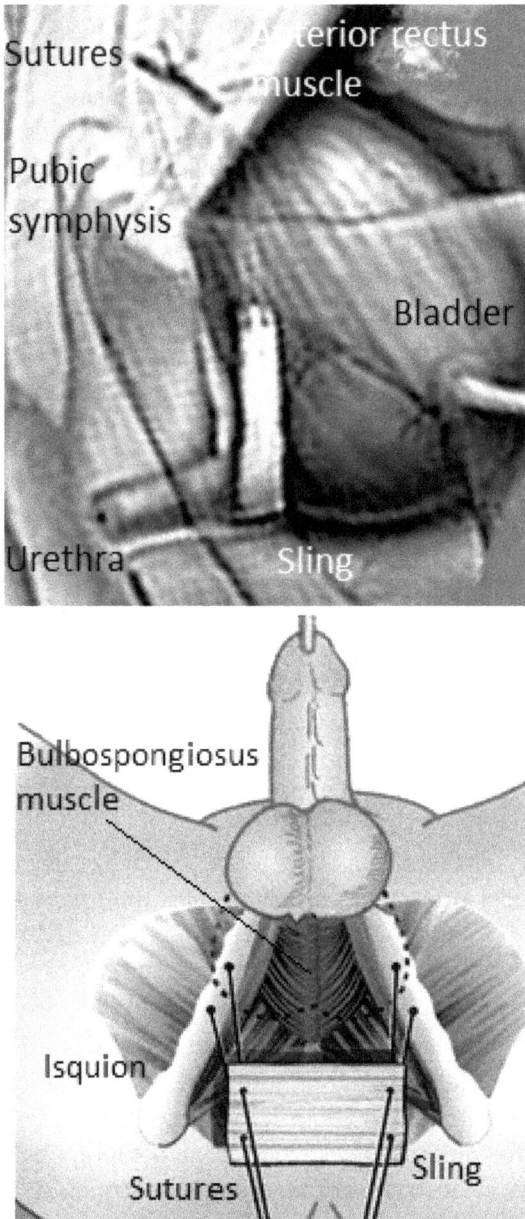

Fig. 46. Autologous patch sub urethral sling. Top female, bottom male.

In men the slings are placed via a retro-scrotal approach and compress the bulbar urethra.

— Peri-urethral injections: they aim is to create a peri-urethral compression effect (Fig. 47). This increases urethral closure pressure by the submucosal injection of bulking, non-reactive substances. Bulking agents used include: dextranomer, hyaluronic acid, autologous fat, tetrafluroethylene (Teflon®), silicone, collagen, pyrolytic carbon, etc. This is a minimally invasive technique, easy to perform, but with mediocre long term results. It often needs repeating, with additional cost being the main inconvenience.

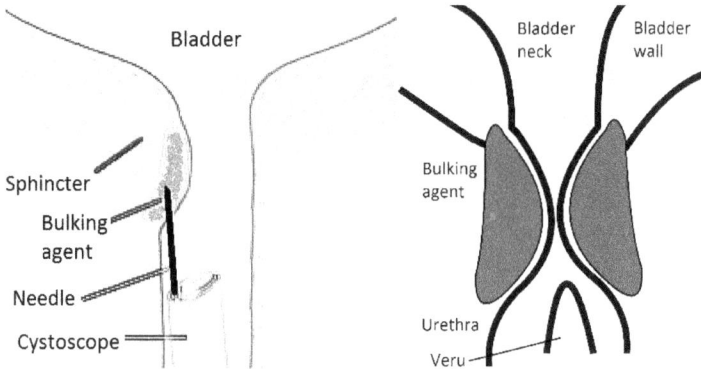

Fig. 47. Female and male bulking agent treatment.

Consider peri-urethral bulking agents (silicone, carbon beads or hyaluronic acid + dextrane co-polymer) for the treatment of SUI if conservative treatment has failed. Patients need to be aware that:
- They may need repeated injections to obtain a result.
- Efficacy tends to wear off with time.
- Efficacy is inferior to either autologous or synthetic slings.

An alternative method of injection is via a suprapubic approach, passing the cystoscope through the sheath of a suprapubic placement kit (SUSIT, suprapubic urethral sphincter injection therapy). This avoids urethral disturbance and leaves a suprapubic catheter so the treated area remains at rest during the early recovery days (Fig. 48).

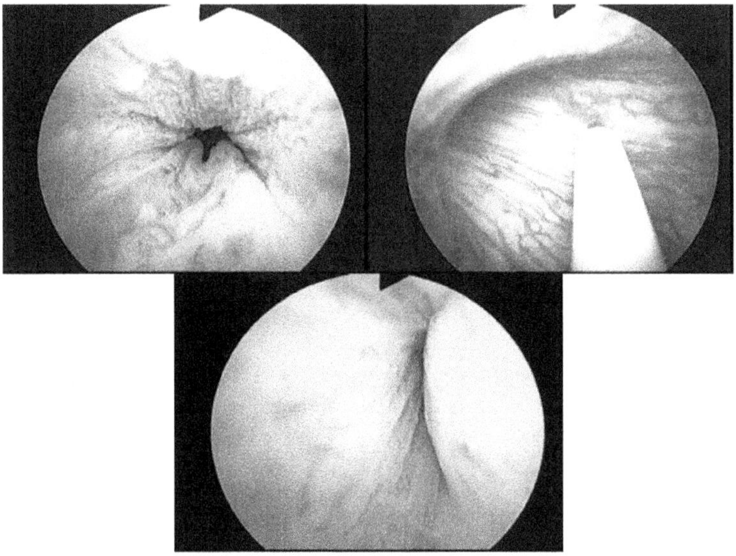

Fig. 48. Suprapubic antegrade injection (SUSIT).

— Artificial urinary sphincter: it requires patients capable of operating it correctly. It can be used in selected neuropathic patients, male post prostatectomy urethral damage, and very exceptionally in SUI in females where all other alternatives have failed. It consists of an inflatable cuff that is placed around the urethra or bladder neck. This cuff is inflated with fluid during the filling phase. It is deflated with a valve, located in the scrotum or labia majora when the patient needs to void. At that time the fluid goes to a reservoir placed in the retro pubic space of Retzius (Fig. 49).

As with other surgical procedures, incontinence operations have better results when performed by surgeons and centres with a high caseload. Twenty procedures or more seem a reasonable number, with less than 5 annual cases requiring some sort of clinical support.

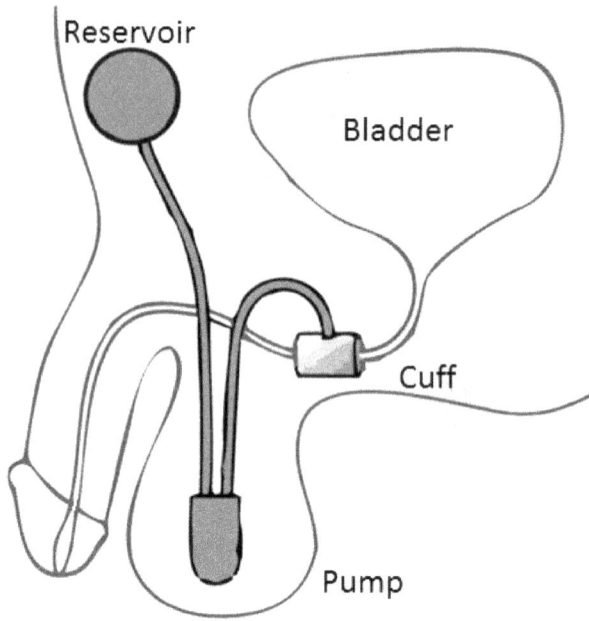

Fig. 49. Artificial urinary sphincter.

MIXED URINARY INCONTINENCE.

It's best to start with behavioural, dietary and hygiene treatment measures and then progress on to medication at least for 4 to 8 weeks. At this point, the patient outcomes can be re-assessed and the residual symptoms assigned to OAB or SUI. With this information and with urodynamic studies if needed, a more invasive treatment plan can then be formulated.

ENURESIS.

Enuresis is UI during sleep. The term is usually applied to the condition in children over 5-6 years as described in the section on development.

Types of enuresis:
• Primary enuresis: there have never been dry nights for a period greater than six months. Its aetiology is unknown and although inheritance plays an important role in this type of enuresis, it has no prognostic value or influence in treatment.
- Monosymptomatic enuresis: the only urinary symptom is urine leakage during sleep.
- Non-monosymptomatic enuresis: there are night leaks and other symptoms such as: incontinence, urgency, etc., during the day.
• Secondary enuresis: enuresis appears after a dry period of at least six months. Always investigate the cause. It can be secondary to emotional problems, patients with constipation, pinworm infestation and obstruction of the upper airway. Rarer causes include diabetes mellitus or insipidus.

Factors involved in the pathophysiology of enuresis include: genetic, hereditary, urodynamic (decreased bladder capacity, overactive bladder, voiding dysfunction), hormonal (impaired release of vasopressin), abnormal sleep pattern, psychological, psychiatric, constipation, sleep apnoea, diabetes, allergy and bacteriuria.

To assess the type of enuresis always obtain a full history and voiding diary and rule out neuropathic dysfunction with a focused physical examination:
• Abdominal examination, and ruling out a palpable bladder.
• External genitalia looking for congenital defects. Wet or soiled underwear.
• Inspection of the back and spine looking for signs of dysraphism.
• Gait observation.

A study with children aged 5-15 years has shown that enuresis is associated with a weaker attachment to the mother, lower patient self-esteem in all areas (affective, bodily, school and family) and more emotional problems, hyperactivity, behavioural disturbances and problems with peers than controls. This theoretically could be avoided with an adequate and early treatment of enuresis. Treatment should start early to improve the child's low self-esteem and avoid a negative impact on the patient and family.

Do not routinely start treatment before 5 years old. Explain the family that positive reward systems for an adequate behaviour must be used either alone or combined with other enuresis treatments. For example rewards can be given for: drinking adequate amounts of fluids at the correct times, voiding before going to sleep, participating in management (like taking the prescribed medication or changing bed clothing).

A positive response to an intervention is considered when the child can achieve 14 consecutive dry nights or a 90% improvement in the number of dry nights over a period.

Given the complexity of enuresis aetiology, treatment can be approached in several ways:

— **The treatment with the highest success rate is an enuresis alarm.** It is a conditional behavioural technique (bed alarm) trying to train the child to retain their urine or wake them up with the alarm that goes off when the pad is wet. This makes the child aware of the unconscious voiding; helping him/her to try to postpone it, and do it in an adequate place (Fig. 50).

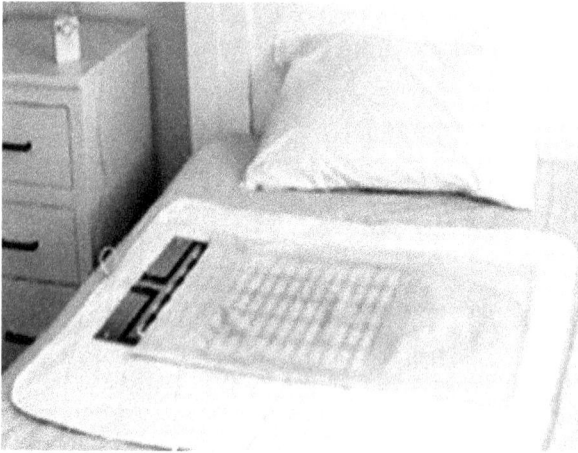
Fig. 50. Enuresis alarm.

—Medication: the elective products are anti-diuretic hormone (ADH) analogues, like Desmopressin, that produces an effective reduction of night time urine production. It's available as tablets and inhaler. Dose is 200-400 mcg/d oral before bedtime. It produces early results, but there are recurrences when discontinued.

Imipramine, a tricyclic anti-depressant is effective due to both its anticholinergic and sympathic effects on the bladder wall. It also helps via making sleep lighter and an increase in ADH production. Dose is 25 mg in less than 8 years and 50 mg in older children. Anticholinergics are more useful when there is detrusor over activity or daytime symptoms of OAB.

The response rate to medications is good, but recurrences tend to be high when medication is stopped. Therefore it is advised to combine them with other strategies.

— Fluid control: enuretic children should consume their fluids during the day; bring forward their last meal and avoid drinking afterwards. They benefit from delaying for 2 or more hours the time after their last meal and going to sleep. They also must empty their bladders before going to bed. These simple measures require family cooperation, and changing daily routines and habits, so they are sometimes neglected.

— Success and failure calendar, where the child registers dry and wet nights. This helps boost self-esteem with successes and involve the child in his/her own treatment. Use a big calendar in a visible place for the child. There are mobile phone applications available for this too.

— Avoid using pads. These are seen as "safety devices" that interfere with the aim of cure.

—Reassure the whole family to **avoid anxiety**, particularly reminding them of the >90% spontaneous remission rate by puberty.

—Other treatment options: acupuncture, PTNS and biofeedback.

ADDITIONAL READING.

1. Guía de práctica clínica: Enuresis nocturna primaria monosintomática en Atención Primaria. Úbeda Sansano M., Martínez García R., Díez Domingo J. Rev Ped At Prim. 2005; 7:61-3.
2. An epidemiological study of nocturnal enuresis in Taiwanese children. Chang P., Chen W.J., Tsai W.Y., Chiu Y.N. BJU Int. 2001; 87(7):678-81.
3. Epidemiology of childhood nocturnal enuresis in Malaysia. Kanaheswari Y. J Paediatr Child Health. 2003; 39(2):118-23.
4. DSM-IV: Manual diagnóstico y estadístico de los trastornos mentales (1994). American Psychiatric Association. Valdés Miyar M, (ed.). Barcelona: Masson; 2001.
5. Standardization and definitions in lower urinary tract dysfunction in children. International Children's Continence Society. Norgaard J.P., van Gool J.D., Hjalmas K., Djurhuus J.C., Hellstrom A.L. Br J Urol. 1998; 81(Suppl 3):1-16.
6. Clinical efficacy and safety of desmopressin in the treatment of nocturnal enuresis. Klauber G.T. J Pediatr. 1989; 114(4 Pt 2):719-22.
7. Annotation: Night wetting in children: Psychological aspects. Butler R.J. J Child Psychol Psychiatry. 1998; 39(4):453-63.
8. Child psychiatry aspects of enuresis nocturna. Von Gontard A. Wien Med Wochenschr. 1998; 148(22):502-5.
9. You feel helpless, that's exactly it: Parents' and young people's control beliefs about bedwetting and the implications for practice. Morison M.J., Tappin D., Staines H. J Adv Nurs. 2000; 31(5):1216-27.
10. Voiding habits and wetting in a population of 4,332 Belgian schoolchildren aged between 10 and 14 years. Bakker E., Van Sprundel M., Van der Auwera J.C., van Gool J.D., Wyndaele J.J. Scand J Urol Nephrol. 2002; 36(5):354-62.
11. An Italian epidemiological multicentre study of nocturnal enuresis. Chiozza M.L., Bernardinelli L., Caione P., Del Gado R., Ferrara P., Giorgi P.L., et al. Br J Urol. 1998; 81(Suppl 3):86-9.

12. An epidemiological study of primary nocturnal enuresis in Chinese children and adolescents. Wen J.G., Wang Q.W., Chen Y., Wen J.J., Liu K. Eur Urol. 2006; 49(6):1107-13.

13. Prevalence of enuresis in 4-to-16-year-old children: An epidemiological study. Verhulst F.C., van der Lee J.H., Akkerhuis G.W., Sanders -Woudstra J.A., Donkhorst I.D. Ned Tijdschr Geneeskd. 1985; 129(49):2260-3.

14. The epidemiology of childhood enuresis in Australia. Bower W.F., Moore K.H., Shepherd R.B., Adams R.D. Br J Urol. 1996; 78(4):602-6.

15. Nocturnal enuresis: a survey of parental coping strategies at 7 1/2 years. Butler R.J., Golding J., Heron J. Child Care Health Dev. 2005; 31(6):659-67.

17. Nocturnal enuresis at 7.5 years old: Prevalence and analysis of clinical signs. Butler R.J., Golding J., Northstone K. BJU Int. 2005; 96(3):404-10.

16. Nocturnal enuresis and overactive bladder in children: An epidemiological study. Kajiwara M., Inoue K., Kato M., Usui A., Kurihara M., Usui T. Int J Urol. 2006; 13(1):36-41.

17. Differences in characteristics of nocturnal enuresis between children and adolescents: a critical appraisal from a large epidemiological study. Yeung CK, Sreedhar B, Sihoe JD, Sit FK, Lau J. BJU Int. 2006; 97:1069-73.

18. Psychological correlates of enuresis: a case-control study on an Italian sample. Coppola G, Costantini A, Gaita M, Saraulli D. Pediatr Nephrol. 2011; 26:1829-36.

19. Nocturnal enuresis in children: prevalence, correlates, and relationship with obstructive sleep apnea. Su MS, Li AM, So HK, Au CT, Ho C, Wing YK. J Pediatr. 2011; 59:238-42.

20. Examination of the structured withdrawal program to prevent relapse of nocturnal enuresis. Butler RJ, Holland P, Robinson J. J Urol. 2001; 166:2463-6.

21. Oral desmopressin: a randomized double-blind placebo controlled study of effectiveness in children with primary nocturnal enuresis. Skoog SJ, Stokes A, Turner KL. J Urol. 1997; 158:1035-40.

22. The efficacy and safety of oral desmopressin in children with primary nocturnal enuresis. Schulman SL, Stokes A, Salzman PM. J Urol. 2001; 166:2427-31.

OVERFLOW INCONTINENCE.

In patients with voiding dysfunction, the obstruction needs to be treated to resolve retention. Overflow incontinence is a complete urinary retention and needs to be managed as such. Incontinence here is just a symptom.

In children with functional voiding dysfunction and incontinence, biofeedback can help. With the adequate equipment, the child is made aware of physiological mechanisms that are not conscious, so he/she can modulate them and try to normalise them. The better responders are children with poor voiding coordination (inadequate striated sphincter relaxation during voiding, non-neurogenic or behavioural dyssynergia).

URINARY FISTULAE.

Fistula means an abnormal communication between two epithelial surfaces. Fistula frequency is reducing due to advances in medical treatments and better healthcare. Although infrequent, this type of incontinence must be identified, prevented and treated.

Uro-genital fistulae.

1. Vesico-vaginal fistulae.
   These are the most prevalent fistulae. In underdeveloped countries, obstetric trauma is the main cause of these complications, followed by caesarean sections and uterine ruptures. In 8% of cases there are associated recto-vaginal fistulae or third degree perineal muscle tears. In developed nations, gynaecologic surgery is the most frequent cause of vesico-vaginal fistula (VVF). Abdominal or vaginal hysterectomy is associated with 75% of them (Fig. 51a). Previous uterine surgery, endometriosis, and pelvic radiotherapy are predisposing factors. Congenital anomalies, infections, foreign bodies and locally advanced pelvic tumours are responsible of non-iatrogenic fistulae.

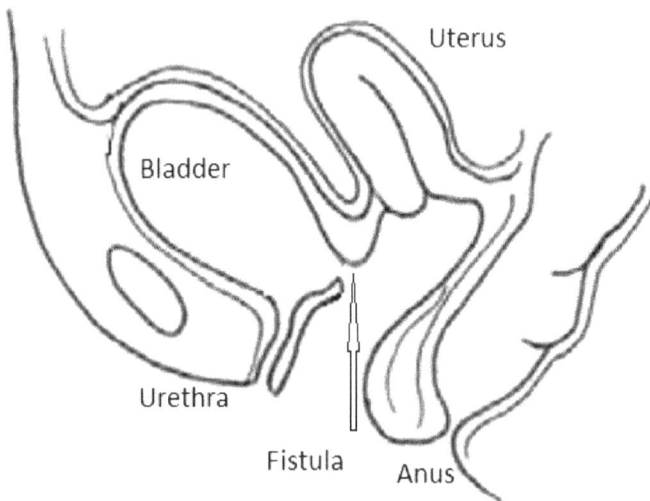

Fig. 51 a. Vesico-vaginal fistula.

AETIOLOGY:

Congenital.

Acquired:

1. **Iatrogenic**
   a) Hysterectomy
   b) Incontinence surgery
   c) Anterior colporrhaphy
   d) Pelvic laparoscopy
   e) Gynaecologic biopsies
   f) Radiation damage

2. **Non-iatrogenic**
   a. Advanced pelvic carcinoma
   b. Traumatic vaginal delivery
   c. Infectious- tuberculosis
   d. Foreign bodies (vaginal or vesical)

A patient can present with continuous urine leakage through the vagina between the first and second postoperative weeks after a pelvic operation. Suspicion can be also raised by a torpid postoperative recovery, lower abdominal pain, paralytic ileus, OAB or haematuria. Incontinence, which is usually total and permanent, is the classical sign of this condition. Radiation fistulae can present months or years after treatment, and must be interpreted as recurrent cancer until proven otherwise by biopsy. Pelvic examination and diagnostic manoeuvres must confirm that the aqueous liquid from the vagina is urine, confirm that the leakage is not coming through the urethra, and if possible, localize the fistulous orifice location.

Differential diagnosis include incontinence due to detrusor or urethral dysfunction, ureteral ectopy, urethro-vaginal fistula, urinary uterine fistula, vaginal discharge of peritoneal fluid, Fallopian tube fistula, infectious vaginitis and pelvic abscess.

High urea and creatinine in the fluid can confirm that it is urine. The patient must be assessed by means of cystoscopy and full vaginal examination. Cystoscopy will localize the lesion and relate it to the ureteral orifices, size, number of fistulae and maximum bladder capacity, as well as any other associated problems.

Vaginal examination must assess the inflammation and induration of the vaginal wall. In cases of previous tumours and/or radiotherapy, biopsies are needed to confirm recurrence. For all these reasons, it's usually better to perform these studies under general anaesthetic.

It is mandatory to assess the upper urinary tract, since in 10% of these patients there is an associated uretero-vaginal fistula. CT is the most frequent technique used, but retrograde pyelography is more reliable, and can be done during the cystoscopy.

A properly done voiding urethro cystogram will show the fistulous tract and contrast in the vagina, as well as other associated problems like cystocele, urethral failure, urethro-vaginal fistulae, and vesico-ureteral reflux. MRI provides excellent diagnostic images, in several planes and without exposure to ionizing radiation, and should be done as the single and comprehensive study when available.

Urodynamic studies are contraindicated, since, as always, the anatomical defect must be repaired before a functional study can be entertained. Intravenous urogram is a historical study with no advantage over the previously described imaging modalities.

To try to minimize the physical and psychological impact of a VVF an early repair has to be considered. A bladder catheter, urethral or suprapubic should be used to reduce urine leakage before surgical repair. It's also paramount to plan the rational use of antibiotics to control possible bacterial and mycotic infections. In postmenopausal patients, HRT improves vascularization and the general quality of the tissues. Repair success rest on the approximation and closure of tissue layers without tension, with no inflammation and with the best possible vascularization. The timing of repair depends on each case, but the resolution of inflammation of the peri-fistulous tissues is the limiting factor.

In small fistulae, < 5 mm, without ischaemia, radiation, or inflammation, a trial of continuous bladder drainage can be attempted, preferably by a suprapubic catheter. Antibiotics should be used to keep urine as sterile as possible.

Anticholinergics will reduce detrusor contractions. This scheme can see up to 10% of small post-hysterectomy fistulae close.

Most fistulae can be repaired through a transvaginal approach, which is less invasive than an abdominal one and leads to a quicker recovery. The technique consists in the creation of an inverted "U" shaped vaginal flap on the anterior wall, multilayer, no tension closure and the adequate use of well vascularized overlapping flaps. In some cases ureteral stenting will be needed, as they facilitate the creation of these flaps and exposure of the defect.

Abdominal access is reserved for patients with complicated or complex fistulae, need for ureteral re-implantation or augmentation cystoplasty. Repair success with both approaches range between 85 and 100%. Post radiotherapy fistulae or recurrent cancer may require colpocleisis or urinary diversion.

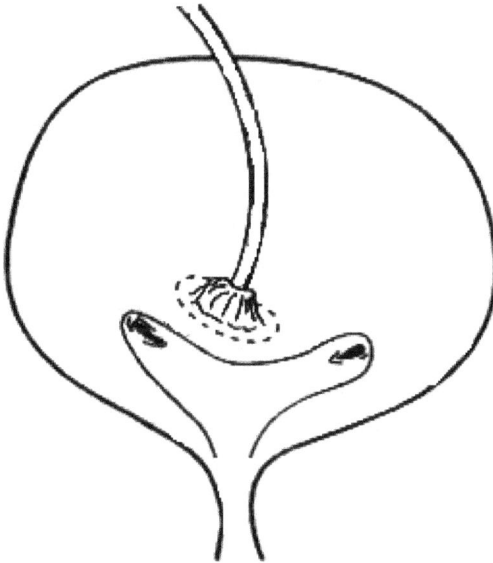

Fig. 51b. Sub-peritoneal transvesical abdominal approach. Fistula tract catheterised with Foley/Fogarty balloon catheter. Traction is used to resect or dissect the edge of the fistula. Followed by closure in 3 or 4 layers (vagina, fascia, detrusor, and mucosa) that are non-overlapping to try to avoid suture line overlay.

Fistulae repair access:

VAGINAL:

    Advantages:
- a) Less invasive
- b) Quicker recovery
- c) Shorter surgical time
- d) Not necessary to open the bladder
- e) Lower cost

    Disadvantages:
- a) Smaller surgical field
- b) Limited access, especially in narrow vaginas
- c) Cannot address associated abdominal, ureteral and some bladder problems

ABDOMINAL:

    Advantages:
- a) Good exposure
- b) Possibility to address associated abdominal, ureteral and some bladder problems

    Disadvantages:
- a) More invasive
- b) Slower recovery
- c) More expensive

Techniques for fistulae repair:

I) ENDOSCOPIC TECHNIQUES:
- a) Endoscopic treatment by injection of fibrin glue or collagen (high failure rate, minimally invasive, for very small fistulae <3mm).
- b) Laparoscopic access and repair with any required procedure.

II) OPEN TECHNIQUES:
- a) Abdominal approach (for atrophic vaginas or the need to use abdominal tissues). (Fig. 51b).
- b) Vaginal approach (for good trophism and accessible defects). (Fig. 52).
- c) Combined approach (complex defects).

III) FLAP INTERPOSITION (do it whenever possible):
   a) Martius labial fat pad (distal lesions).
   b) Gracilis muscle or mio-cutaneous flap (extensive defects, including post-radiotherapy).
   c) Omentum or peritoneal fat (abdominal approach).
   d) Peritoneal flap (trans-vaginal approach).
   e) Anterior abdominal rectus muscle (extensive defects, including post-radiotherapy).

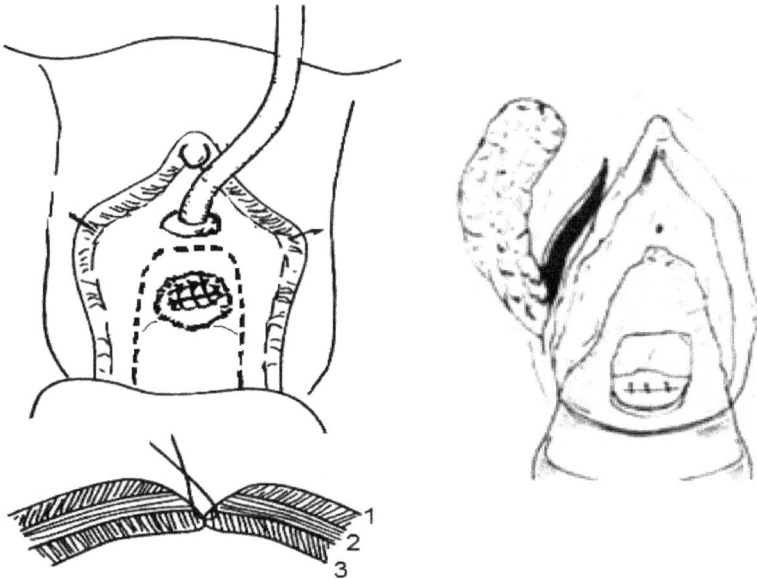

Fig. 52. Vaginal approach. Urethra catheterized with Foley catheter. Inverted U shaped incision of the vaginal wall. Closure in 3 or 4 layers (vagina -3-, fascia -2-, detrusor and mucosa -1-) non-overlapping to try to avoid suture line overlay. The vaginal wall flap (thin line) is advanced to the external and superior edge close to the urethral meatus to finally close the vaginal wall. Martius labial fat flap on left.

2. Urethro-vaginal fistulae.
    Urethro-vaginal fistulae have a similar aetiology to VVF. In developed countries they're associated with pelvic surgical procedures whilst in developing countries obstetric complications are the main cause. Fistulae affecting the middle and distal thirds of the urethra, below the sphincter area can be asymptomatic or

101

produce a urine flow that is partly vaginal (hypospadic meatus). Fistulae of the proximal third of the urethra produce constant leakage or SUI. The assessment of these defects requires evaluation of the extension of the lesion, presence of urethral hypermobility, intrinsic sphincter deficiency (ISD) and trophism of vaginal tissues. Uretrhoscopy with a 0 degree lens and a no beak cystoscope can identify the fistula, the extension and associated problems in the trigone and bladder neck. VCUG is a useful tool and must show frontal and lateral views. Surgical repair follows the same general principles than VVF. Most repairs are done transvaginal, with the abdominal approach reserved for patients with trigonal and bladder neck compromise or requiring ureteral re-implantation.

3. Vesico-uterine fistulae.
An acquired communication between the uterus and the bladder is infrequent and usually associated with obstetric complications. Accounts for 3% of uro-genital fistulae and in more than half of the cases is secondary to a caesarean section. It can also happen after long labour, forceps deliveries and uterine ruptures. The clinical scenario will depend on the length and direction of the fistulous tract, and particularly, its relation to the uterine isthmus. An isthmus fistula, is usually one way, from the uterus to the bladder, and can present with cyclical menstrual haematuria and amenorrhea. Here the patient is continent due to the tone of the isthmus. Fistulae below the isthmus produce incontinence, isolated or mixed with menstrual bleeding, as urine can go both ways. Clinically they can present as incontinence (50 to 85%), cyclical menstrual haematuria and amenorrhea or a combination of both. Sometimes urine leakage can be seen from the cervix orifice with stress manoeuvres. VCUG can show contrast in the uterine cavity. As before, MRI is the imaging tool of choice, and can detect and follow the fistulous tract.

For surgical repair, an abdominal, subperitoneal, transvesical approach or a transperitoneal alternative are the preferred routes. In post-menopausal patients or patients not wishing further children a hysterectomy is usually done.

4. Uretero-vaginal fistulae.

The relation of the pelvic ureter with the female genital tract facilitates the lesion of the distal ureter during pelvic and retroperitoneal gynaeco-obstetric procedures. Uretero-vaginal fistulae produce permanent incontinence, independent of stress manoeuvres. Gynaecological surgery is the cause of most of these lesions with a 1.6% incidence. Simple hysterectomy accounts for 60% of them. Other contributing procedures include: adnexal surgery, anti-incontinence surgery and anterior vaginal wall surgery. Urology, digestive, vascular and orthopaedic procedures can also damage the ureters. Independently of the mechanism of damage, a defect is created in the ureter wall with urine leakage, which either accumulates into a collection or more often finds a way to the vagina, peritoneum, uterus, intestines or skin. There is a significant local inflammatory reaction that will later lead to ureteral stenosis. These fistulae present with incontinence with or without normal voiding. The patient can also have pain in the compromised side of the pelvis, and occasionally an urinoma can be palpated. The ureter lesion leads to postoperative pain and torpid postoperative recovery, obstruction and dilatation of the compromised urinary system, nausea, vomits, abdominal distention, paralytic ileus, fever, malaise and finally incontinence. The vaginal fluid is confirmed urine by the elevated creatinine and urea levels when compared with plasma. Chromoscopy can be done by injecting indigo carmine i/v and filling the bladder with methylene blue whilst the vagina is packed. Green indigo carmine will lead to a ureter fistula, while methylene blue will be seen in VVF or urethro-vaginal fistulae when the packing is removed. Renal function needs to be assessed. MRI and CT will show upper tract dilatation in 90% of cases and the fistulous tract. They also provide information on renal function, uni- or bilateral compromise, level and size of defect(s) and associated lesions. (Fig. 53). Aetiology can occasionally be identified. Imaging assists to plan the repair by showing the relation between the ureter and the vagina as well as the other pelvic organs. Multi-plane imaging and 3D reconstruction are useful as well. A retrograde pyelogram during the cystoscopy can confirm diagnosis and help plan treatment, it also allows for ureter stenting, which is part of the endoscopic treatment. Ultrasound scanning is of limited value other than identifying dilatation and bladder capacity.

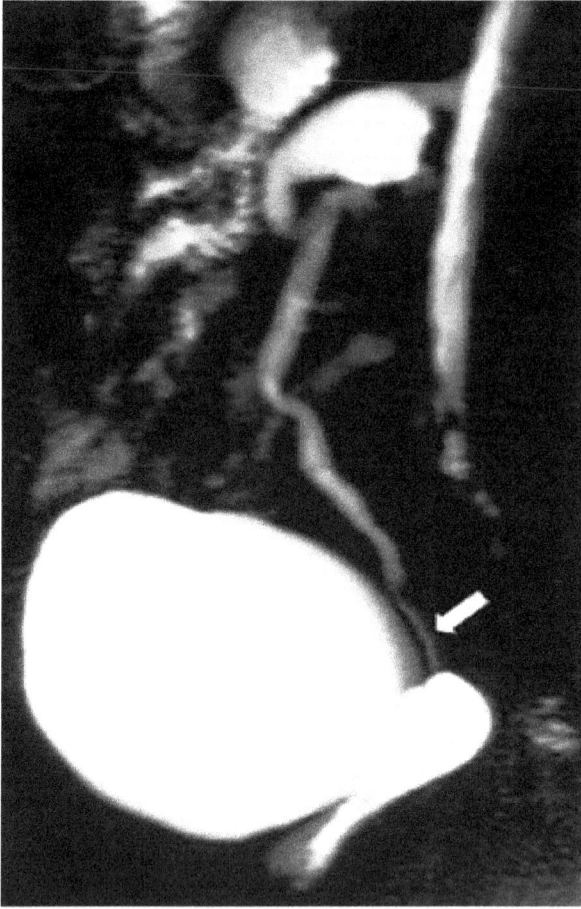

Fig. 53. MRI confirms uretero-vaginal fistula. Lateral view.
Proximal dilatation is seen.[xii]

Crushing lesions can be managed by JJ stenting for 4 weeks. If there is ischaemia or direct lesion, a mobilisation, spatulation of both ends and end to end anastomosis over a JJ stent is done. Ureter stenting is essential for adequate drainage and healing, as it keeps ends aligned, and drainage prevents obstruction above the anastomosis produced by oedema. A nephrostomy can be used as an initial measure, to drain the involved system until inflammation resolves for an elective repair. Antegrade contrast studies can also provide useful imaging.

If the ureter wall is only partially damaged a JJ stent is usually corrective.

If an endoscopic procedure is not possible or has failed, open repair is the standard. The need for a non-tension anastomosis limits the use of a uretero-ureterostomy to discrete lesions of the medial or upper ureter. Distal ureter lesions are better managed by ureter re-implantation. To assist with a non-tension re-implantation a psoas hitch (bladder mobilization and lateralization by suturing to the psoas muscle) or a Boari flap (bladder-wall base flap) can be used, and they can cover gaps up to 15 or 20 cm. In more complex situations a trans-uretero-ureterostomy, segmental ileal substitution or auto transplantation can be considered. A nephrectomy is rarely needed nowadays.

Uro-cutaneous fistulae.
Kidney to skin tracts are the result of surgical or endoscopic procedures, more rarely from stone and/or infectious disease.

Vesico-cutaneous fistulae are more frequent in males, usually as a consequence of prolonged suprapubic catheterisation or any other surgical procedure that can compromise the anterior vesical wall. Predisposing factors include infra-vesical obstruction and detrusor over activity.

Urethro-cutaneous fistulae are usually a sequela of urethral surgery, peri-urethral infection or any complicated urethral stricture.

The clinical picture includes leakage by a skin orifice that can be permanent or intermittent. The patient generally has an associated infection with variable systemic compromise.

Here again MRI and CT are the more reliable tests to assess the fistula, identify the underlying abnormalities and show the anatomical relation between the affected organ and the fistula. A contrast CT can also provide an idea of split renal function. A VCUG will provide similar information as in vaginal fistulae, and so will the cystoscopy that can accurately obtain biopsy samples.

Urethro-cutaneous fistulae can drain through the perineum and they will evolve according to the associated presence of strictures. With inflammation and obstruction there may be multiple tracts that tend to appear with elevated pressures and infection. VCUG and urethroscopy are key diagnostic tools.

Pyelo-cutaneous fistulae are managed by JJ stenting and a urethral catheter, reducing system pressure to zero. Up to 20% may require nephrectomy. Surgical repair stands on removing any obstruction, preserving renal function, debridement of compromised tissues, interposition of well vascularized ones and adequate drainage.

Most urethro-cutaneous fistulae are a consequence of failed hypospadias repairs. The surgical solution includes multilayer closure with flaps if necessary, and trying to avoid superposition of suture lines. Patients will require suprapubic drainage to allow for adequate healing, and any strictures must be dealt with.

PALLIATIVE TREATMENTS.

When there is no curative solution for incontinence, there are alternative strategies which may suit the patient's needs and allow them to lead as normal a life as possible. This allows for social integration of the patients and avoids the hygienic consequences of incontinence. Some of the devices used include: indwelling catheters, collecting devices and bags, occlusion devices for the urethra, and absorbent products.

— Indwelling catheters: these are a last resource in continence provision for the long term. They're also used as a temporary measure during treatment of ammonia dermatitis and decubitus ulcers. They can be urethral or suprapubic (better tolerated). (Fig. 54). Unless there is a formal contraindication (like autonomic dysreflexia), indwelling catheters should be used closed with a valve. This allows for bladder filling, and bladder emptying when deemed convenient (by opening the valve). This type of use has the transcendent function of avoiding a non-functional, small and atrophic bladder that leads to serious complications.

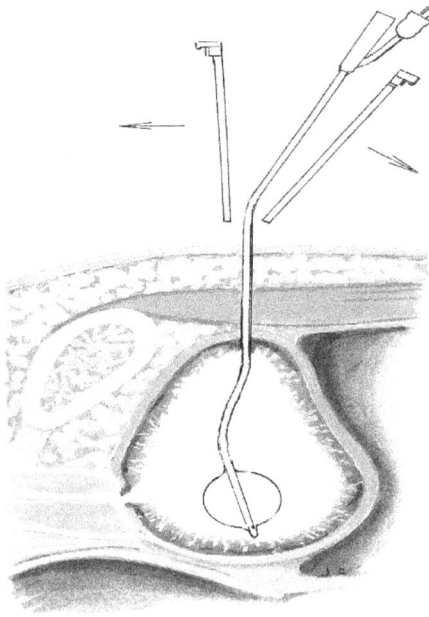

Fig. 54. Suprapubic cystostomy.

— Collecting sheaths: these devices are condom-like and end in a tube that allows connection of a standard urine collecting bag. (Fig. 55). They should never be applied so tight that would produce penile compression, as this can lead to erosion and fistulae, particularly in patients with sensory deficits.

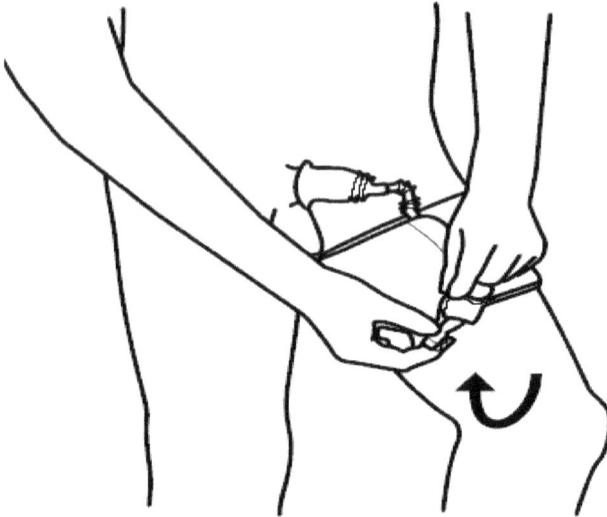

Fig. 55. Collecting sheath.

— External occlusive devices: these are slings or clamps that are placed around the penis generating compression that closes the urethra. They are rarely used due to poor effectiveness, discomfort and high likelihood of penile skin lesions (Fig. 56 A and B).

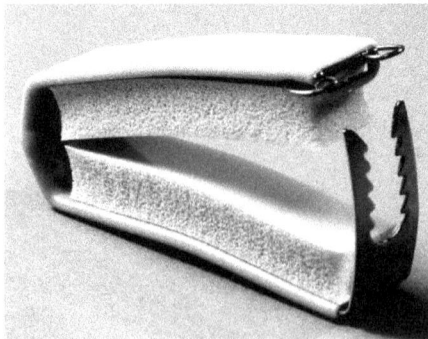

Fig. 56 A. Penile clamp.

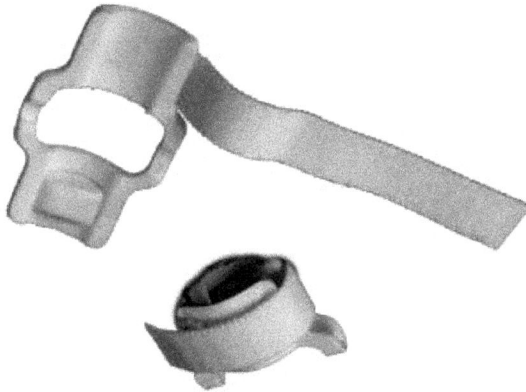

Fig. 56 B. Penile compression device.

— Urine collection bags: these store urine in a discrete way. Some are designed to be adhered around a stoma, whilst others are connected to a catheter or external collector sheath.

— Absorbent devices: these are the most frequently used palliative devices for incontinence. They are usually disposable and are used in contact with the body to absorb and retain urine in them. This keeps the skin relatively dry. Every incontinent person can use absorbent products as these are non-invasive and easy to use. Depending to their design and absorption capacity they can be used for mild to severe incontinence. The selection of the absorbent product will depend on the patient's needs, diuresis, and daytime or night time use. Absorption products are made of several layers:

1) filtration layer, which is in contact with the skin. It's made of hydrophilic porous material that allows for quick passage of urine to the centre of the device, keeping the skin dry.

2) absorption centre, this is made of cellulose and an absorption material. The urine is held by the molecules of the absorbent substance/gel, and becomes solid. This prevents the urine to spill back to the skin or outside the device.

3) external waterproof layer, this prevents dampness to pass to the clothes. This usually has a dampness indicator that indicates when urine reaches this layer and the garment needs changing (Fig. 57).

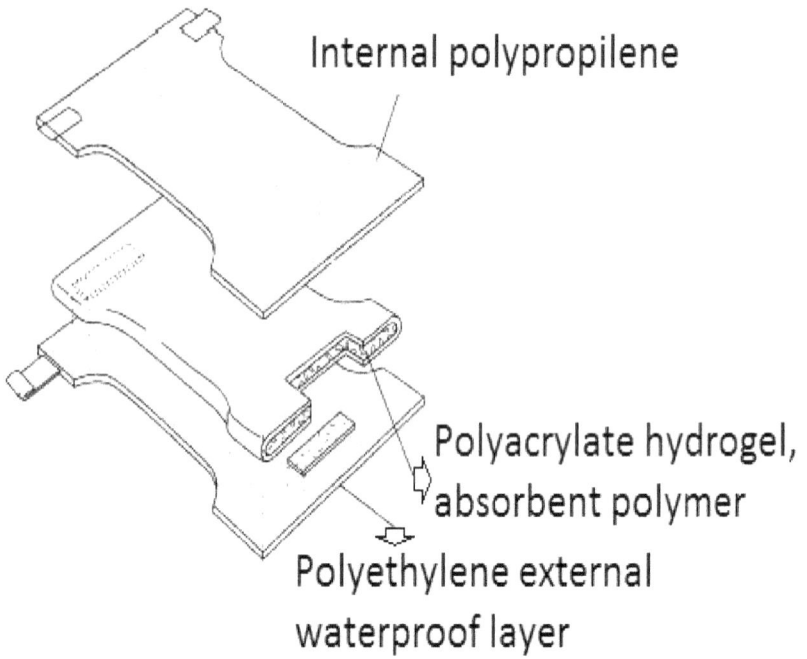

Fig. 57. Absorbent products layers.

ADDITIONAL READING.

1. Ten-year experience with transvaginal vesicovaginal fistula repair using tissue interposition. Eilber KS, Kavaler E, Rodríguez LV, Rosenblum N, Raz S. J Urol. 2003 Mar; 169(3): 1033-6.
2. Incontinencia urinaria. Incontinencia urinaria en las personas mayores. Ruiz Cerda JL, Martínez Agulló E, Burgués Gasión JP, Arlandis Guzmán S, Jiménez Cruz JF. Doyma Newsletter; 2002; 5: 1-12.
3. Enuresis persisting into adulthood. Shadpour P, Shiehmorteza M. Urol J. 2006. Summer; 3(3): 117-29.
4. Tratamiento de la incontinencia post prostatectomía con estimulación eléctrica perineal. Martínez L, Lorenzo L, Malfatto G, Clavijo J, Decia R, Machado M. 1er Congreso de Urología del MERCOSUR. Punta Del Este. Uruguay. 2001.
5. Outcomes of Suprapubic Urethral Sphincter Injection Treatment (SUSIT) for Stress Incontinence in Women. Rajbabu K, Clavijo Eisele J, Lawrence W. Congress of the European Society for Urological Research. Athens. 2004.
6. Urinary incontinence. NICE Guideline. 2020.
7. Difference of opinion - Are synthetic slings safe? Opinion: No. Ackerman AL, Raz S. Int Braz J Urol. 2016 Jul-Aug; 42(4): 640-4.
8. Guidelines on Urinary Incontinence. European Association of Urology. 2020.
9. Giggle incontinence: micción patológica durante la risa. Fernández, W., Clavijo, J. Lab. de Neuro-urología. Depto. de Urología. Hosp. de Clínicas. Montevideo. I Congreso Ibero-Americano de Neuro-urología y Uro-ginecología. Punta Del Este. Uruguay. 1989.
10. Minimally invasive polypropylene mesh sling for stress incontinence. Clavijo-Eisele J, García L. J. Endourol. Vol. 15 (Supl 1), V6-P1, 2001.
11. Incontinencia urinaria y Urología femenina. Reporte de Beca de la Confederación Americana de Urología. Clavijo-Eisele J. Dep. of Urology. UCLA Medical Center. Los Angeles. US. 1997.
12. Detrusor myectomy: long-term functional outcomes. Aslam MZ, Agarwal M. Int J Urol. 2012 Dec; 19(12):1099-102.
13. The treatment of adult enuresis and urge incontinence by enterocystoplasty. Bramble FJ. Br J Urol. 1982 Dec; 54(6): 693-6.
14. Fístulas urinarias. Puesta al día. Allona Almagro A, Sanz Migueláñez JL, Pérez Sanz P, Pozo Mengual B, Navío Niño S. Actas Urol Esp. 2002 Nov-Dec; 26(10): 776-95.
15. Male perineal sling with autologous aponeurosis and bone fixation - description of a technical modification. Rios LA, Tonin RT, Panhoca R, De Souza OE, Filho L, Mattos D Jr. Int Braz J Urol. 2003 Nov-Dec; 29(6): 524-7.
16. Percutaneous Tibial Nerve Stimulation (PTNS) efficacy in the treatment of lower urinary tract dysfunctions: a systematic review. Gaziev G, Topazio L, Iacovelli V, Asimakopoulos A, Di Santo A, De Nunzio C, Finazzi-Agrò E. BMC Urol. 2013 Nov 25; 13:61.
17. Urodynamic evidence of effectiveness of botulinum A toxin injection in treatment of detrusor overactivity refractory to anticholinergic agents. Kuo, HC. Urology 2004; 63: 868.
18. Vesicouterine fistula. A review. Tancer, M.L. Obstet Gynecol. Surg. 1988; 41:743.
19. Urological complications of pelvis radiotherapy. Solsona E. y colab. En Jewett MAS; Ed Oxford: Isis Medical Media; 1995:51.
20. Surgical repair of vesicovaginal fistulas. Huang. W.C. y colab. Urol. Clin. N. Amer. 2002; 29 (3) 709.

21. Early repair of iatrogenic injury to the ureter or bladder after gynecological surgery. Blandy J.P. y colab. J. Urol. 1991; 146:761.
22. Transvaginal repair of vesicovaginal fistula using a peritoneal flap Raz, S. y colab. J. Urol. 1993; 150:56
23. Observation on prevention and management of vesico-vaginal fistula after total hysterectomy. Tancer M.L. Surg. Gynecol. Obstet 1992; 175:501.

CHAPTER 5. NEUROPATHIC BLADDER.

Rosenbaum T and Clavijo J.

CONTINENCE MANAGEMENT OF PATIENTS WITH NEUROPATHIC BLADDER.

Neurologic lesions can produce a permanent and constant deficit in the nervous system (like a CVA, SCI or cauda equina compression) or a progressive one (dementia, Parkinson's disease, MS, peripheral neuropathy).

Fig. 58. Some neurological diseases that can affect the function of the lower urinary tract:

	Congenital and peri-natal diseases	"Stable" diseases	Progressive or degenerative diseases
Central nervous system	Cerebral palsy	CVA Encephalic lesions	Multiple sclerosis. Parkinson's disease. Dementia. Multisystem atrophy.
Supra sacral spinal cord	Spinal dysrraphysm (myelomeningocele, etc.)	Spinal cord injuries	MS. Cervical spondylosis.
Sacral spinal cord and peripheral nerves	Spinal dysrraphysm. Sacral Agenesis. Ano-rectal anomalies.	Cauda equina syndrome. SCI. Pelvic nerves damage secondary to radical pelvic surgery.	Peripheral neuropathy.

Cerebral lesions produce an interruption of the connection paths between the cerebral cortex and the pontine micturition centre, and consequently the loss of voluntary control of the filling/voiding cycle. When the bladder is full, it will contract by the medullary reflex loop. The patient will have no control of this even if he/she is aware of the voiding sensation and the ensuing incontinence.

Supra-sacral lesions are located between the PMC and the spinal centres. These lesions will affect the thoracic and cervical spine. The nuclei in the unaffected sections are not damaged and the reflexes work, but they are disconnected from the PMC, where coordination between bladder and sphincter happens. If the spinal injury is complete, the bladder becomes automatic, with reflex emptying when full. The patients usually don't have voiding sensation. Since the spinal centres are not connected to the PMC, no input is received in the PMC, and no output is sent to relax the striated sphincter. This is called detrusor-sphincter dyssynergia (DSD). Dyssynergia results in a sustained detrusor contraction with a closed bladder neck and closed striated sphincter that lead to high intravesical pressures and functional obstruction.

The proximity of the neurological areas that control the digestive system and sexual response with the area that controls continence and voiding means that many patients with neurological problems will have a combination of urinary, digestive and sexual dysfunctions. The clinical team must address these problems not in isolation but trying to provide the best possible global solution.

Symptoms of neurogenic urinary tract dysfunction can be related to continence or voiding. Storage symptoms include frequency and incontinence. The patients can also present with symptoms related to complications like urinary infections, stone disease or renal failure. These may present differently in patients with neurologic impairments.

Treatment usually does not restore normal urinary function and quality of life can be affected by the treatment itself. Patients often have to endure medications' side effects, the social and psychological consequences of self-catheterisation, the impact of a long term catheter and the permanent use of medication or devices. All these also impact family and carers, who may have problems with the physical demands required to care for a neurological patient with urinary problems, and face social and psychological challenges.

Preserving renal function is of paramount importance. Renal failure is the main cause of mortality in patients with SCI that survive the initial insult. This led to the golden rule in the management of neuropathic bladders: make sure that intravesical pressure is within safe limits both during filling and voiding phases. This strategy has significantly reduced mortality by urological complications in these patients.

Treatment of urinary incontinence is important for patients' rehabilitation, thus improving their quality of life. It is also crucial to reduce the incidence of urinary infections. When complete continence cannot be achieved, we can use strategies to provide an acceptable social control of incontinence. Patient quality of life is a fundamental part of any treatment decision.

The financial cost of neurogenic urinary dysfunction is considerable. This includes protective pads and garments, appliances, catheters, medication, and surgical procedures. An additional financial burden includes the need for carers, nursing and medical input. The ability of a person to work can be affected by the neurogenic dysfunction. There is also a significant expense for patient follow up, which usually is lifelong.

EVALUATION.
Complete clinical assessment, including urology and neurology physical examination (at least a basic one). Knee (L2-L4) and bulbo-cavernous (L5-S5) reflexes cover most relevant areas. Quality of life should be measured with validated tools (RAND 36 or similar), and re-checked after an intervention. Consider assessing renal function by accurate methods like creatinine clearance or isotope GFR with DMSA or DTPA.

Ultrasound scan.

Offer permanent surveillance with urinary USS to high risk patients for renal complications on an annual basis. This high risk group includes SCI, spina bifida, and patients with urodynamic low compliance, detrusor-sphincter dyssynergia or vesico-ureteral reflux.

Urodynamic studies.
Routine UDS (cystometry and PFS) are not necessary in patients at low risk of renal complications, like most patients with multiple sclerosis.

Organize UDS in high risk patients (SCI, spina bifida, ano-rectal anomalies). Also have updated ones before surgery for neurogenic dysfunction. In high risk patients have UDS done every 2 years or sooner if clinically necessary.

TREATMENT.
Provide information that is adequate to the physical condition and cognitive function of the patient (and/or guardian) to directly involve them in the care and management plan. In patients with high bladder pressure during the filling phase (detrusor hyperactivity/hyper-reflexia, low compliance) or the voiding phase (DSD, other causes of obstruction) treatment is aimed to change a **high pressure bladder in a low pressure reservoir, in spite of residual urine, which can be emptied by intermittent catheterisation**. This is a vital concept that must be kept in mind at all times.

Non-invasive treatment.
Assisted bladder emptying: incomplete bladder emptying (and therefore residual urine) is a significant risk factor for UTIs, high bladder pressure during the filling phase, deterioration of renal function and incontinence. In neuropathic bladder dysfunction (NBD) patients use several methods to improve the emptying process.

- Voiding through abdominal strain (Valsalva) or hypogastric compression (Credé) must not be used as they produce high bladder pressures. Patients must be warned of this risk.

- Triggered reflex voiding: sacral or lumbar dermatomes stimulation in patients with spinal lesions can produce a reflex detrusor contraction. It's unusual that this contraction is coordinated with a sphincter relaxation and of low pressure. It therefore must not be used unless it has been found safe when elicited during a urodynamic study. Patients must be warned of this risk.
- Cognitive behavioural techniques (CBT): they're used to improve continence and include immediate voiding, programmed or timed voiding (bladder drill) and modification of life habits.

Medication: there is no single medication to treat NBD. A combination of adequate and individualized medications is the best way to optimize results. Anticholinergics are still the most used drugs to manage NDO. Neuropathic patients usually require a higher dose than the one used for idiopathic DO. Mirabegron, a selective beta 3 agonist is the usual second line medication approach in patients without contra-indications.

Phosphodiesterase inhibitors (PDE5i) like Sildenafil showed significant effects on detrusor over activity and in the future may become an alternative or addition to other detrusor relaxant medications.[xiii]

The selective addition of Desmopressin or Imipramine can increase treatment efficacy.

Detrusor under activity: the use of cholinergic medications such as Betanecol chloride or Distigmine bromide does not produce any effective detrusor contraction during voiding attempts. Therefore do not use them and inform the patient of the risks of incomplete emptying.

Increase of resistance of the urethral closure system: several compounds have shown efficacy in selected cases of mild stress urinary incontinence. Side effects can be serious in patients with NBD. Do not routinely use them and warn the patient of side effects risks.

Do not offer alpha blockers as treatment for urinary retention (obstruction) due to NBD. They are not effective, as they lead to high bladder pressure during voiding and consequent renal dysfunction. Educate the patient about this risk.

Peripheral tibial nerve stimulation can be used with moderate results but without significant side effects.[xiv]

Intravesical electrical stimulation can be of some use in selected patient with reduced detrusor contraction to assist in voiding with effective pressures.

External devices: as a last resource, social continence can be achieved by collecting the urine during incontinence. Penile sheath collectors (condom like) are a practical method for males. Otherwise absorbent products can offer a viable solution. In both cases vigilance is needed due to the risk of infection. Due to the risk of producing elevated bladder pressure, penile clamps are contraindicated (and they also produce skin lesions).

In catheterised patients, for UTI prevention, assess the possibility of use of a flow valve, spigot or close the catheter as an alternative to continuous drainage into a collecting bag. Consider patient, family and carer's preferences, as well as manual dexterity, cognitive capacity and lower urinary tract function of the patient (Fig. 59).

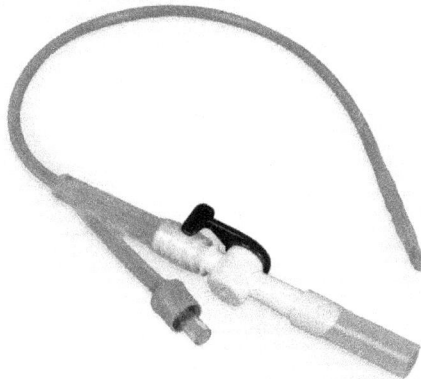

Fig. 59. Catheter with valve.
Intermittent catheterisation.

Intermittent catheterisation (IC) by the patient or by a carer (assisted) is the management method of choice for NBD. It's effective in patients with:

- Underactive or non-contractile detrusor.
- Detrusor hyperactivity (hyperreflexia) once treated.

Sterile IC reduces significantly the risk of bacteriuria and UTIs compared with clean IC. However the former is not the usual management, use it in immune suppressed patients or whilst in hospital only. Clean (aseptic) IC is an alternative that produces a beneficial effect regarding reduction of external contamination. Daily frequency is 4 to 6 times, and the catheter size 12 to 14 Fr. Doing it less frequently leads to higher volumes and increased risk of UTIs. More frequent ones increase the risk of external contamination and UTIs and traumatic complications. Bladder volume before IC should be 400 ml or less. Complications are reduced by patient education, atraumatic technique, and basic hygienic precautions to prevent UTIs (Fig. 60 and 61).

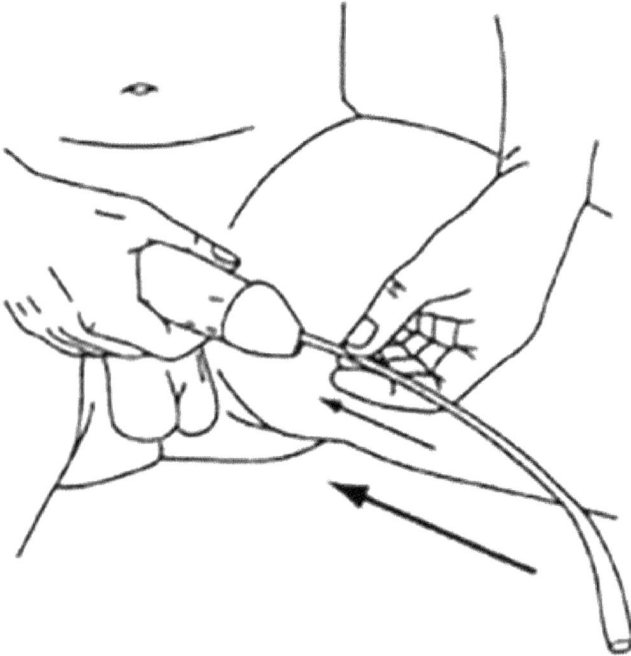

Fig. 60. Self-catheterisation, male.

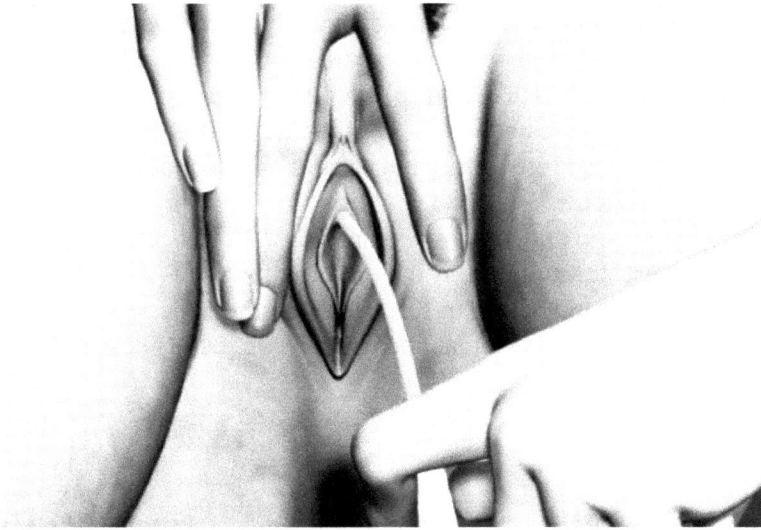

Fig. 61. Self-catheterisation, female.

Permanent catheterisation.
A permanent urethral catheter, and to a lesser extent a suprapubic cystostomy catheter are early and important risk factors of UTIs and other complications (stone, cancer). Silicone catheters are the preferred ones as they are less likely to calcify and due to the high latex allergy in patients with NBD. Permanent urethral or suprapubic catheterisation should only be used exceptionally, under strict control, and catheters should be changed with their ideal frequency. Silicone catheters can be changed every 4 to 6 weeks, whilst latex ones need more frequent replacement. Silver coated catheters can last up to 3 months or more. Change frequency can vary according to local microbiology situation and guidance.

Endoscopic treatments.
Intravesical pharmacological treatment (resiniferotoxin) has unreliable results so can only be entertained in a research protocol.

Intravesical injections of botulinum toxin: botulinum toxin A produces a reversible chemical denervation that last 6 to 12 months. The injections are applied to the bladder wall in a dose adequate to the formulation used. Botulinum toxin A has been shown efficacious in a randomized controlled trial versus placebo in NBD. Generalized muscle weakness is an occasional adverse side effect. Standard dose is 200 to 300 IU. Botulinum toxin injection in the bladder wall is the more effective minimally invasive treatment to reduce neurogenic detrusor over activity.

Botulinum toxin A injections with intermittent self-catheterisation is the best treatment for the vast majority of patients with hyperreflexia and a urethral closure system at least moderately competent. The injection technique has been described in previous chapters.

Surgical treatment.
Urethral and bladder neck interventions.
The increase of the urethral closure system resistance has the risk of leading to high bladder pressures during voiding (obstructive uropathy). Interventions to treat sphincter incontinence are only safe and useful when detrusor function is controlled (or normalised) and there is not a significant vesico-ureteral reflux. These techniques require the urethra and bladder neck to be in good condition and most of them will require intermittent catheterisation after the procedure.

These interventions include urethral suspension with slings in females. In males, slings are less predictable and an artificial urinary sphincter (AUS) is the most frequent option. In patients with neurogenic stress incontinence avoid synthetic slings. The AUS has passed the test of time even in the challenging neurogenic patients. The need for revision has been reduced with newer devices. The technique has been described above.

Sphincterotomy and bladder neck incision result in incontinent patients and should not be used routinely.

Bladder interventions.
Detrusor myectomy: this has acceptable to modest results on the long term. Advantages include: low surgical morbidity, low incidence of adverse effects on the long term, positive effect on patients' quality of life, and it does not significantly increase the risk of future interventions (Fig. 62).

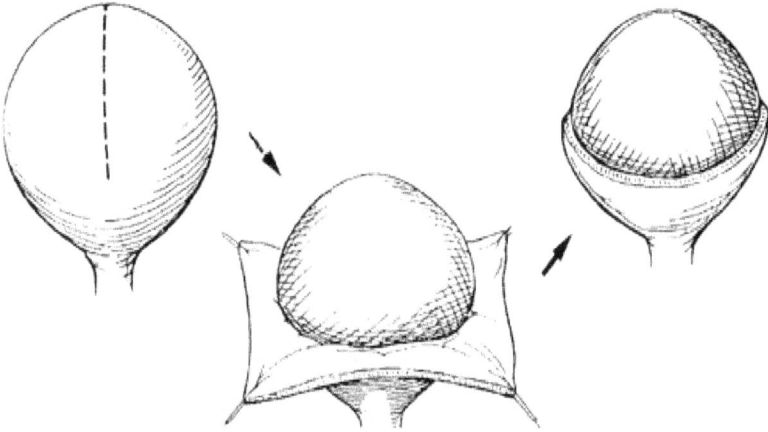

Fig. 62. Auto-augmentation by detrusor incision and bladder mucosa expansion (wide mouth diverticulum-like).[xv]

Denervation, afferent nerve/root section, neuro-stimulation and neuromodulation: these diverse techniques are aimed to interrupt or modify bladder nerve supply and function. They have been largely abandoned or selectively restricted due to their poor or too variable results on the long term and some severe complications. Sacral anterior roots stimulation, with or without rhizotomy, as described by Brindley can benefit highly selected patients, with occasional coordinated voiding and reasonable pressures. The role of standard sacral root stimulation is still undefined[xvi].

Augmentation cystoplasty.
Consider this procedure using a de-tubularized intestinal section patch in patients with non-progressive neurological conditions and without urinary complications (like upper tract dilatation) and only after a complete clinical and urodynamic assessment. The patients and/or carers and family must be aware of possible complications, the risks and alternative options. These patients will require lifelong follow up after cystoplasty due to the long term risk of complications. Potential complications include metabolic imbalances, like vitamin B12 deficiency and bladder stones and cancer.

Effects of bladder augmentation: bladder capacity expansion with intestine (or more rarely a neo-bladder) will eliminate or reduce detrusor hyperreflexia. Complications include: UTIs, stones, perforation, patch metaplasia or cancer, metabolic changes, mucus production and short bowel syndrome. Since the age of the patients having the operation is lower than those who have it for bladder cancer, it is relevant to consider longer term complications. Therefore this procedure should be used with caution in neurogenic patients, but it can be necessary when all other less invasive options have failed.

Augmentation cystoplasty is a valid option to reduce bladder pressure and increase bladder capacity. Several techniques have been described, and the most frequently used has already been described in the urge incontinence chapter.

Urinary diversion.
When no other treatment has been successful or possible, a urinary diversion can be considered to protect the upper urinary tract and improve the patient's quality of life.

Continent diversions: these should be the first option. It is a better option than a permanent urethral catheter or a suprapubic one. Some patients with limited manual dexterity prefer a stoma rather than using the urethra for intermittent catheterisation, particularly females. A continent stoma can be fashioned in several ways. All have frequent complications like necrosis, peri-ostomal hernia, or stenosis. Short term continence is over 80% and the upper urinary tract is well protected. For several reasons, including cosmetic, the umbilicus is usually the place to locate the stoma (Fig. 63).

Incontinent urinary diversion: when intermittent catheterisation is not viable or impossible (visual or dexterity impairments, carers' issues) an incontinent diversion can be fashioned with the stoma connected to a collecting bag. Fortunately, the indication for this procedure is infrequent nowadays, as there are several better and adequate alternatives.

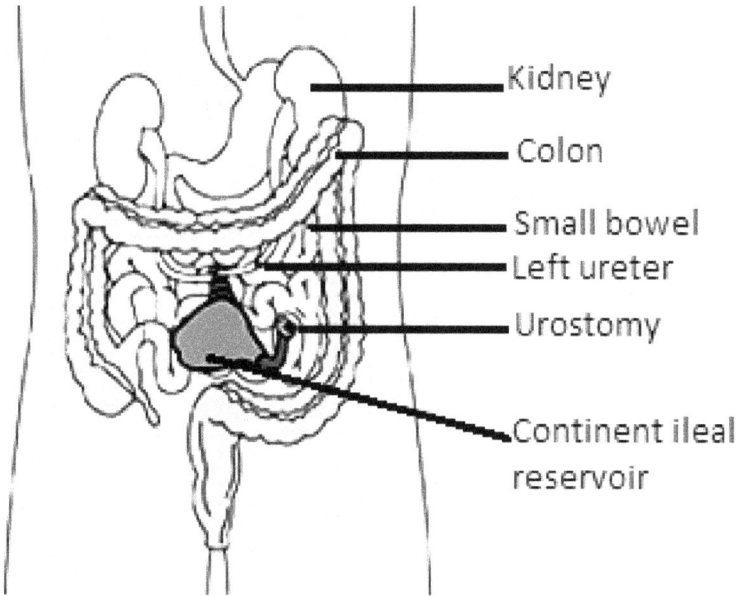

Fig. 63. Continent ileal pouch with cateterizable stoma.

This procedure can be considered in patients, who are wheelchair bound or bedridden with intractable and incontrollable incontinence, patients with very poor bladders, when the upper urinary tract is compromised and in patients who refuse other options. In most of the cases an ileal conduit is used (Fig. 64). Long term results are poor and the foreseeable complications demand a permanent follow up. The urinary diversion can be done with a simple cystectomy to avoid the complications of a non-functioning excluded bladder.

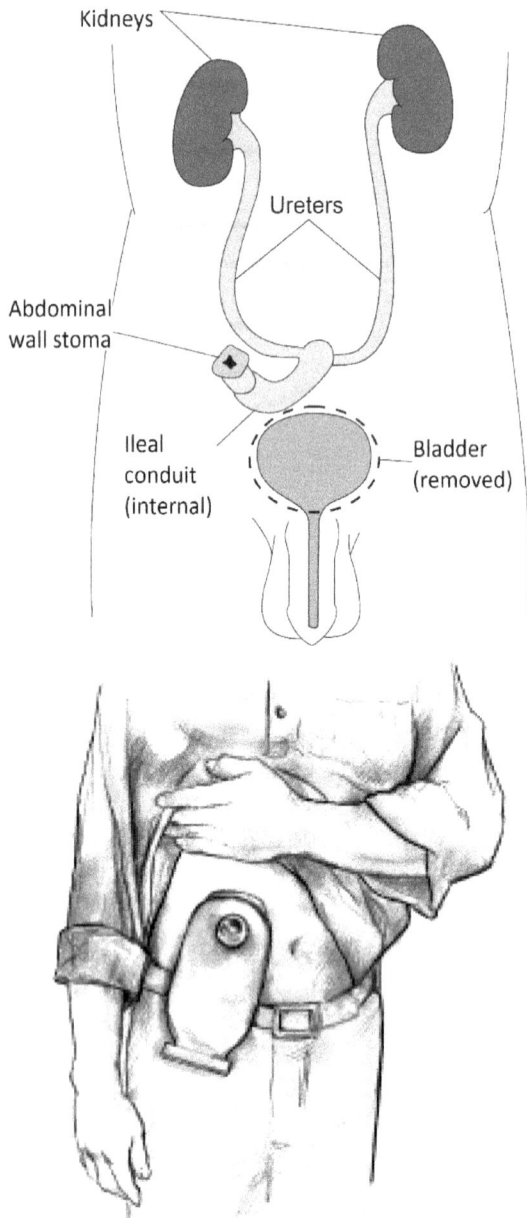

Fig. 64. External incontinent urinary diversion with an ileal conduit, with or without cystectomy.[xvii]

AUTONOMIC DYSREFLEXIA.

Definition.
Autonomic dysreflexia (AD) is a massive unregulated autonomic sympathetic reflex response in patients with spinal cord injury (SCI) above the sympathetic level (T5-T6).

It is a rare but dangerous medical emergency characterised by a sudden elevation in blood pressure which requires immediate action. Clinician alertness is essential as SCI patients usually have no sensation or pain below the spinal cord level lesion.

Aetiology.
The nerve supply of the viscera is the autonomic nervous system which emerges from the brain stem and spinal cord at higher levels than the corresponding somatic nerves. All autonomic activity becomes disconnected from the somatic activity below the level of the cord injury.

A sensory input (generally not perceived due to the neurological lesion) usually from bladder or bowel, produces in the spinal cord a reflex with the output being a segmental sympathic release. This leads to peripheral vasoconstriction and consequent hypertension. The baroreceptors in the carotid arteries detect the hypertension. The brain reacts by reducing the heart rate through the parasympathic system (as far down as it can go due to the SCI). This bradycardia is insufficient to lower the blood pressure, and the hypertension continues. The sympathic autonomic response prevails below the level of SCI, and the parasympathic autonomic response prevails above it.

Frequency is 48-90% of all individuals who are injured at T6 and above. AD occurs during labour in approximately two thirds of pregnant women with SCI above the level of T6. Very careful monitoring and treatment is therefore clearly mandatory.

Diagnosis.
The diagnosis is clinical.

History: any stimulus below the level of the spinal injury can cause an episode of AD (pain and other sensations are obviously abolished below that level). (Fig. 65).

<u>Possible triggers to look for:</u>
- Bladder distention
- Urinary tract infection
- Cystoscopy
- Urodynamics
- Detrusor-sphincter dyssynergia
- Epididymitis or scrotal compression
- Bowel distention
- Bowel impaction
- Gallstones
- Gastric ulcers or gastritis
- Invasive testing
- Haemorrhoids
- Gastro-colic irritation
- Appendicitis or other abdominal pathology
- Menstruation
- Pregnancy (especially labour and delivery)
- Vaginitis
- Sexual intercourse
- Ejaculation
- Deep vein thrombosis
- Pulmonary emboli
- Pressure ulcers
- Ingrown toenail
- Burns or sunburn
- Blisters
- Insect bites
- Contact with hard or sharp objects
- Temperature fluctuations
- Constrictive clothing, shoes, or appliances
- Fractures or other trauma
- Surgical or diagnostic procedures
- Pain (if some nociceptive sensation is preserved)

Symptoms:
- Profuse sweating, especially in the face, neck, and shoulders.
- Goose bumps.

- Flushing of the skin especially in the face, neck, and shoulders; this is a frequent symptom.
- Blurred vision and spots in the visual field.
- Nasal congestion, a common symptom.

Past medical history: previous episodes of AD. Ongoing medical problems.

Physical examination: sudden, significant rise in systolic and diastolic blood pressure.

Signs:
- Abdomen: look for bladder distension, abdominal distension, pressure ulcers, and signs of acute abdomen.
- PR for bowel impaction and haemorrhoids.
- External genitalia: epididymitis, scrotal compression, turbid or offensive urine suggestive of urinary tract infection.
- PV: menstruation, pregnancy, vaginitis.
- Legs: deep vein thrombosis, pressure ulcers, ingrown toenail.
- Generally: burns or sunburn, blisters, insect bites, fractures or other trauma. Profuse sweating above the level of lesion, especially in the face, neck, and shoulders; rarely occurs below the level of the lesion. Goose bumps above, or rarely below, the level of the lesion. Flushing of the skin above the level of the lesion, especially in the face, neck, and shoulders; this is a frequent sign.

Investigations:
Blood: routines including cultures and pregnancy test. FBC for infections.

Urine: dip and cultures (urinary tract infection).

Imaging: ultrasound scan may show bladder distension, gallstones, deep vein thrombosis. X rays and CT scan if fractures or other trauma are suspected.

If information is available from previous urodynamic studies: presence of detrusor-sphincter dyssynergia.

AUTONOMIC DYSREFLEXIA

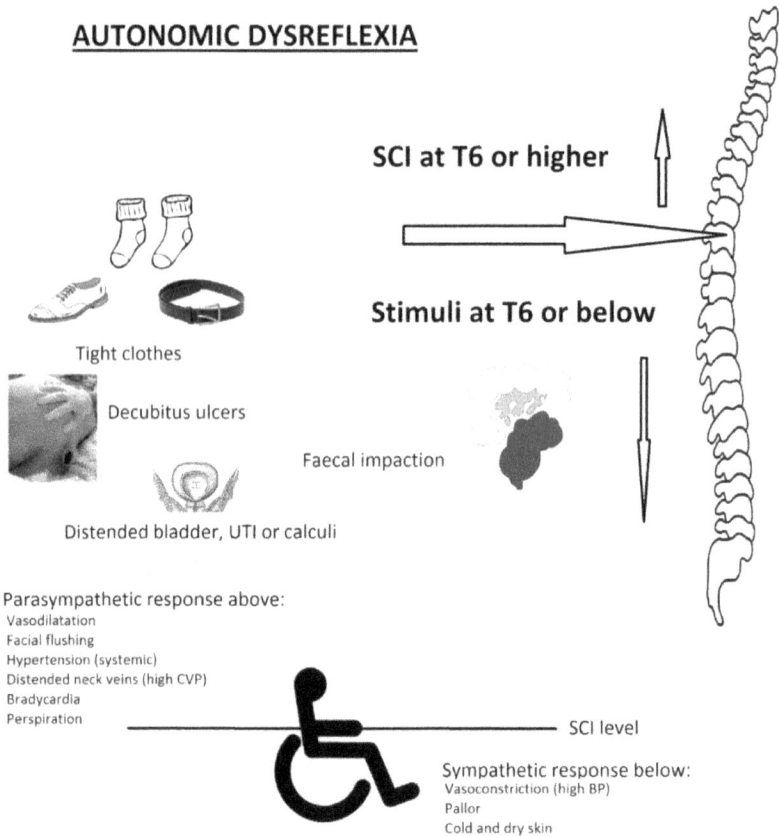

SCI at T6 or higher

Stimuli at T6 or below

Tight clothes

Decubitus ulcers

Faecal impaction

Distended bladder, UTI or calculi

Parasympathetic response above:
Vasodilatation
Facial flushing
Hypertension (systemic)
Distended neck veins (high CVP)
Bradycardia
Perspiration

SCI level

Sympathetic response below:
Vasoconstriction (high BP)
Pallor
Cold and dry skin

Fig. 65. Autonomic dysreflexia trigger stimuli.

Treatment.
Medical.
Sit up the patient immediately and loosen any clothing or constrictive devices. Sitting leads to pooling of blood in the lower extremities and may reduce blood pressure.

If an indwelling urinary catheter is not in place, catheterize the patient. If the patient has an indwelling urinary catheter, check the system along its entire length for kinks, folds, constrictions, obstructions and for correct placement.

Use an antihypertensive agent with rapid onset and short duration while the causes of AD are being investigated if the blood pressure is at or above 150 mm Hg systolic. The most commonly used agents are Nifedipine and nitrates (e.g., Nitroglycerine). Nifedipine should be in the immediate release form; bite and swallow is the preferred method of administering the drug, not sublingual administration.

Patients who have previously experienced episodes of AD are treated with antihypertensives prior to procedures known to cause this reaction.

Surgical treatment is necessary if there are trigger factors that require it for resolution.

Complications.
Complications associated with autonomic dysreflexia result from severe peripheral hypertension and include retinal and/or cerebral haemorrhage, myocardial infarction, seizures and death.

Outcomes.
Once the initial stimulus is removed, the hypertension resolves.

ADDITIONAL READING.

1. The importance of autonomic dysreflexia to the urologist. Shergill IS, Arya M, Hamid R, Khastgir J, Patel HR, Shah PJ. BJU Int. 2004 May; 93(7): 923-6.
2. Autonomic dysreflexia and its urological implications: a review. Trop CS, Bennett CJ. J Urol. 1991 Dec; 146(6): 1461-9.
3. Autonomic dysreflexia: an important cardiovascular complication in spinal cord injury patients. Gunduz H, Binak DF. Cardiol J. 2012; 19(2): 215-9.
4. Autonomic dysreflexia: a medical emergency. Bycroft J, Shergill IS, Chung EA, Arya N, Shah PJ. Postgrad Med J. 2005 Apr; 81(954): 232-5.
5. Rehabilitation medicine: 1. Autonomic dysreflexia. Blackmer J. CMAJ. 2003 Oct 28; 169(9):931-5.
6. Urinary incontinence in neurological disease: Management of lower urinary tract dysfunction in neurological disease. NICE guideline CG148. August 2012. www.nice.org.uk/guidance/cg148.
7. Guía clínica sobre la disfunción neurógena de las vías urinarias inferiores. M. Stöhrer, D. Castro Díaz, E. Chartier Kastler, G. Del Popolo, G. Kramer, J. Pannek, P. Radziszewski, J J. Wyndaele. European Association of Urology. 2010.
8. Autonomic Dysreflexia. Clavijo J, Rosenbaum T. (2016) pp 197-201. In: Handbook of On Call Urology. 2nd Ed. Urology Solutions Publishing. Lincolnshire. UK. 2016. ISBN: 978-0-9931760-3-6.
9. The first 500 sacral anterior root stimulators: implant failures and their repair. Brindley GS. Paraplegia. 1995 Jan; 33(1):5-9.
10. Transcutaneous electrical nerve stimulation in the treatment of patients with poststroke urinary incontinence. Guo ZF, Liu Y, Hu GH, Liu H, Xu YF. Clin Interv Aging. 2014 May 23; 9: 851-6.
11. Botulinum-A toxin as a treatment of detrusor-sphincter dyssynergia: a prospective study in 24 spinal cord injury patients Schurch B, Hauri D, Rodic B, Curt A, Meyer M, Rossier A. J Urol 1996; 155: 1023.
12. Augmentation cystoplasty in the treatment of neurogenic bladder dysfunction. Linder A, Leach GE, Raz S. J Urol. 1983 Mar; 129(3): 491-3.

Index.

Images.

---

[i]   From www.fvfiles.com.

[ii]   From www.ucla.edu.

[iii]   From www.urospec.com.

[iv]   From wikiHow, Creative Commons License.

[v]   Modified from wikiHow. CCL.

[vi]   From BAUS.org.

[vii]   Modified from Medtronic®.

[viii] Modified from IUGA.

[ix]   Seki N, Shahab N (2011). Dysfunctional Voiding of Non-Neurogenic Neurogenic Bladder: A Urological Disorder Associated with Down Syndrome. In: Genetics and Etiology of Down Syndrome. Prof. Subrata Dey (Ed.). ISBN: 978-953-307-631-7. InTech.

[x]   Plata-Salazar M and Torres-Castellanos L.

[xi]   Modified from DynaMesh®.

[xii]   Mamere A E, Coelho R D, Cecin A O, Feltrin L T, Lucchesi F R, Pinheiro M A L et al . Evaluation of urogenital fistulas by magnetic resonance urography. Radiol Bras. 2008 Feb; 41(1): 19-23.

[xiii] Gacci M, Del Popolo G, Macchiarella A, Celso M, Vittori G, Lapini A, Serni S, Sandner P, Maggi M, Carini M. Vardenafil improves urodynamic parameters in men with spinal cord injury: results from a single dose, pilot study. J Urol. 2007 Nov; 178(5):2040-3.

[xiv]   Eftekhar T, Teimoory N, Miri E, Nikfallah A, Naeimi M, Ghajarzadeh M. Posterior tibial nerve stimulation for treating neurologic bladder in women: a randomized clinical trial. Acta Med Iran. 2014; 52(11):816-21.

[xv]   Ashraf Abou-Elela (2011). Augmentation Cystoplasty in Pre-transplant Recipients, Understanding the Complexities of Kidney Transplantation, Prof. Jorge Ortiz (Ed.), ISBN: 978-953-307-819-9, In Tech.

[xvi]   Martens FM, Heesakkers JP. Clinical results of a Brindley procedure: sacral anterior root stimulation in combination with a rhizotomy of the dorsal roots. Adv Urol. 2011; 2011:709708.

[xvii] Modified from NIDDK.

www.ingramcontent.com/pod-product-compliance
Lightning Source LLC
Chambersburg PA
CBHW062024200326
41519CB00017B/4921